COLON HYDROTHERAPY

The

Professional Practitioner Training Manual

and

Reference Book

By

Richard Knight

ISBN 978 0 9524392 3 3

© Richard Knight 2010

Printed and bound in the United Kingdom

Typeset in Tahoma

Published by
Cross Roads Publications,
16 South Primrose Hill,
Chelmsford,
Essex,
CM1 2RG
UK

t: 07966174466

Dedicated to

Esther

An inspiration, and principled messenger,

for complementary medicine and the helping professions.

Acknowledgements

I wish to extend my deepest thanks to all the many friends and colleagues who have supported me in the preparation of this book. Their help and kindness made possible the finished book. Especially to:

Nelson Brunton, President of the Association of Natural Medicine, Doctor of Naturopathy, an Acupuncturist, and Researcher into anti-ageing treatments, for his personal encouragement, clinical advice, and for having such a profound knowledge of natural therapeutics.

Bridget Main, Homoeopath and Allergy Clinician, for her commitment to detail, unwavering support, and most insightful suggestions.

Paul Phillips, Technical Director, for his enduring patience and guidance in the preparation of several drafts and re-drafts.

Andrew McCulloch, Media and Publicity Adviser, for his proof-reading, professional perusal, and helpful recommendations.

Elizabeth Hughes, Lecturer in Anatomy and Physiology, and Kinesiologist, for checking the integrity of the A & P content and her natural enthusiasm for learning and teaching.

David Goddard, Naturopath, for his respected 'hands-on approach' and honest appraisal of naturopathic principles and clinical choices.

Carol Jones, Homoeopath and Secretary to the ANM, for her unconditional willingness to provide administrative support whenever needed. I also thank my friends and colleagues on the ANM Governing Council.

Miranda Comerasamy, Designer, for her support and peaceful approach to all things.

Richard Franklin, of Arima Publishing, for his support and commitment to this work.

Finally, to **Valerie**, as someone who cares for those most in need. A true example to all 'wish to be' therapists, of commitment to the patient. Thank you for putting up with the late nights and early mornings, and the highs and lows of this small, but we trust, positive contribution to complementary medicine, theory, and practice.

A Note To The Reader

The therapeutic methods and procedures in this book are based upon the training, experience, and research of the author. Given that each person, their situation, and symptoms are unique, the author and publisher suggest Patients check with their Medical Doctor prior to using any of the approaches discussed in this book.

The symptoms described in this book may be indicative of more than one condition. There is potentially, in many treatments, some risk involved. The author and publisher are therefore not responsible for any adverse effects or consequences resulting from the use of any of the procedures, preparations, or suggestions described in this book, whether they be adopted by Practitioners or their Patients.

Colon hydrotherapy is not a medical procedure, however, it is a naturopathic and complementary approach to treatment, and must therefore be regarded as such. Colon hydrotherapy is but one of the many modalities and methods used in our search for wellness and treatment of disease. Given that fact, the information presented in this book is without prejudice, and made with the intention of contributing to the goals of wider public information, the advancement of health education, increasing the awareness of treatment choice, and knowledge of complementary medicine options.

COLON HYDROTHERAPY

The
Professional Practitioner Training Manual
and
Reference Book

Acknowledgements

CONTENTS

Defecation

The Colon

Main Functions

Caecum

Vermiform Appendix

Ascending Colon

Transverse Colon

Descending Colon

Sigmoid Colon

Rectum

Anus

Hepatic and Splenic Flexure

Valves of Houston

Portal Circulation

Venous Drainage

Autonomic Nervous System

Implications for the Colon

Peristaltic Movement

Stool Classification

Colon Transit Time

Size, Shape, and Texture

Colour

Odour

Gas

Foreword

Colon hydrotherapy is an aspect of naturopathy. Naturopathy is a system of medicine that seeks to promote and enable the body's own self-healing mechanisms to function more effectively in their natural search within us for health, wellbeing, and balance. In other words, the body has not only a natural ability to resist disease but also has inherent mechanisms of recovery, self-regulation, and a state of equilibrium, also known as homoeostasis, which is equal to normal health.

The procedures or modalities of naturopathic medicine cover a wide range of techniques and knowledge including: detoxification, fasting, natural dietetics, homoeopathy, skeletal manipulation, herbal remedies, allergy testing, hot and cold compresses, and colon hydrotherapy. This book has been written as a training and reference manual in colon hydrotherapy.

So, what is colon hydrotherapy?

Colon hydrotherapy comes from the ancient system of enemas and is, therefore, essentially **a process of detoxification.** Warm, filtered water, at low pressure is introduced into the colon via the rectum in order to reach the length of the entire colon (1.5 metres long) for the purpose of cleansing the body of toxins, the removal of stubborn and impacted faecal deposits, parasites, (unfriendly bacteria and worms), mucous, gas, the products of putrefaction, and to facilitate effective elimination. The skilled colon hydro-therapist will also utilize other techniques, for example, massage, and the use of pressure points to assist water absorption, flushing, and elimination.

Clearly, as one might expect, some of the core material gathered in this manual will have similarities to other like professional training documents. Each draws upon the same general body of knowledge. However, in addition to covering the necessary core material for the training of competent Practitioners, this book also places particular significance on understanding the actual helping process as well as the philosophy and protocols of natural therapeutics.

New learning is both challenging and enjoyable. It is important that students are involved in monitoring and evaluating their learning and progress, especially when applying new skills and insights. Inspiring students to use their potential in a safe and stimulating environment is obviously the most important task. It is only then that specific individual needs will be 'heard' and met, thus mirroring the climate and ethos of the helping relationship.

Within the following material the terms Helper, Practitioner, and Colon Hydrotherapist, are read and understood as being interchangeable. Also the terms Client, Patient, or Helpee are equally read and understood as being interchangeable.

I extend my personal gratitude to all the Authors, Teachers, Helpers, and Patients who have been in part the source of my own development and learning. Also, the support I have received over many years from colleagues within the Association of Natural Medicine, registered charity.

Few would argue that the helping profession is a simple one. However, many of us joyfully acknowledge the personal satisfaction and rewards we have received from being just a small part of that most essential of all professions.

Richard

Chelmsford, 2009

The Suggested Training Goals and Learning Outcomes for Training Courses in Colon Hydrotherapy

- To provide 'best practice' information and learning in colon hydrotherapy and associated techniques and knowledge.

- To ensure the learning environment is conducive at all times to the achievement of the specific learning goals.

- To select and train only those students who meet the admission criteria and are considered to have genuine motivation and proven ability and aptitude within the helping profession.

- To ensure that upon completion of their training the student is able to demonstrate competence, knowledge, understanding, and the safe care of patients in the procedure and administration of the colon hydrotherapy treatment regime.

- That upon the completion of their studies, graduates will be conversant with the requirements, standards, regulations, and conduct of best practice.

- To provide appropriate levels of support to students and subsequent Practitioners that encourages the need for their ongoing self-monitoring of skill and knowledge levels, to ensure up-to-date practice, and their continuous professional development (CPD).

- To promote colon hydrotherapy and complementary medicine and work with other relevant organizations and individuals to ensure the professional values, ethics, and the best practice which informs our work reflects 'respect for the individual Patient' and the 'Patient's right to self-determination'.

Suggested Code of Ethics for Practitioners

This code of ethics is about the **principles that relate to a Practitioner's responsibility to Patients, colleagues, organizations to which he or she are associated and may be registered by, responsibility to the profession, as well as responsibility to society in general.**

The ethical issues that we encounter as Practitioners are the same as the moral concerns we all have to address and those upon which our laws and values are based. In other words, actions, by virtue of their consequences, are inherently right or good. Thus, the following ethical statements emphasize our obligations to others, respect for their rights and protection, and are intended to aid Practitioners in the maintenance of the highest **standards of conduct and professional practice.**

- Practitioners must focus upon ensuring they give the Patient their undivided attention by putting out of their mind their own problems, issues, personal concerns, and, indeed, problems from the previous Patient, by actively attending to the Patient and placing them 'first'.

- Practitioners must guard against any emotional involvement which may complicate the Practitioner and Patient relationship.

- Practitioners must improve their knowledge and skill on a continuous basis so they are able to provide the very best standard of treatment to the Patient and contribute to the improvement and advancement of colon hydrotherapy, as well as any additional or other chosen therapy.

- Practitioners must consider the Patient according to holistic principles. By this we mean looking at the whole person and not only specific symptoms.

- Practitioners must honour and uphold the Patient's integrity, individuality, privacy, and maintain confidentiality.

- The above statements embrace the notion of personal

difference including race, culture, age, gender, intellectual, and physical, as well as socioeconomic position. In short, the recognition that everyone is unique.

- Practitioners must record case records and clinical findings methodically and without distortion, and take full account of the Patient's right to inspect their own case record.

- Practitioners must consider the value of allopathic practice and recognize the value of other therapies and work with other Practitioners and/or refer Patients to them when it is in the Patient's best interest to do so.

- Practitioners must never exploit the Patient. For example, by misusing their authority to dominate Patients to the detriment of their wellbeing, or, establishing a relationship which is outside of the boundaries of their Practitioner role. For example, asking a Patient to lend them money or to undertake specific tasks in a way that could be exploitative.

- Practitioners must never make claims either verbally or in writing regarding their ability to cure any given disease.

- Practitioners must never misrepresent themselves in any way regarding their training and qualifications which may be misconstrued by Patients as evidence of having an orthodox medical background.

- Practitioners must be aware that adherence to and active promotion of the foregoing code of ethics maintains the good name of the Profession, Practitioner Register, and best serves the needs of Patients.

Suggested Code of Practice for Practitioners

Any profession of worth must operate within a framework or code of practice which reflects its **belief systems and operational principles**. This is necessary in order to inform and assure users of the given service, that is the Patient, of what it is they may reasonably expect, and also to provide a structure for the Practitioner.

In other words the **Code of Practice,** in conjunction with the **Code of Ethics** and the **Philosophy Informing Helping** are to establish standards for helping, and thereby inform and protect those persons seeking help. **Together these Codes are the basis from which a proper and genuine professional practice should operate.**

- The recognition of the Patient's right to express feelings openly as an essential part of the helping process, without the Practitioner discouraging or condemning the expression of feelings.

- The Practitioner will be involved in making evaluative judgements about the attitudes, actions, or feelings discussed or transmitted by the Patient. As a consequence, the Practitioner must adopt a non-judgemental attitude and, in doing so, exclude assigning guilt or innocence to the Patient.

- The Patient has the right to self-determination in making their choices and decisions. The helping process directly involves the Patient in exploring treatment options within the framework of their own capacity and responsibility to make and 'own' those choices.

- The Practitioner has the professional obligation to preserve the confidentiality of the personal disclosures shared by the Patient. Therefore, 'treating with confidence' means not revealing any information through any public medium which could lead to the identification of the Patient

- The Practitioner must ensure appropriate privacy is afforded to the Patient, as well as sensitivity to all matters associated with modesty.

- The Practitioner must assume full responsibility for their personal hygiene, safe working practices, clean clothing, sterile gloves, and infection control.

- Towels and gowns and any other items used in treatment must be clean and in good repair, and where appropriate be sterile.

- Surfaces must be cleaned and disinfected before and after each Patient, in particular, areas subject to soiling. For example, couch, door knobs, toilet seat, flush handle, and taps.

- Disposable specula and piping must be used and discarded safely, including other items, for example, incontinence pads, gloves, couch paper, or other throwaway soiled articles.

- Faecal matter, blood, vomit, and bodily fluids pose a serious health risk and must be cleaned-up immediately using disposable gloves, bleach, and appropriate disposal. (Disinfectants do not sterilize. Bleach must be used for dealing with spillages of bodily fluid; detergent and hot water for general cleaning and wiping down. Use disinfectants for cleaning the colon hydrotherapy machine and wiping down all other surfaces in the treatment area). The floor of the treatment area must be provided with a smooth impervious surface or covering. The local Environmental Health Department must be advised within 24 hours of learning of any infections or complications arising from any colon hydrotherapy procedure.

- Colon hydrotherapy machines must be fitted in accordance with the instructions of the manufacturers, be fitted with a suitable water filter, be equipped with non-return valves in order to protect the water supply, and there must be a mechanical break between the mains water supply and the Patient. The temperature of the water coming through the speculum should normally be between 33 and 40 degrees centigrade (92° to 104° Fahrenheit) and must never be exceeded.

- The treatment area must be used solely for treatments and have a constant supply of hot and cold water and a wash basin for the Practitioner's own use.

- A toilet, wash basin, and a waste bin for sanitary towels and soiled articles must be available, during working hours, for the Patient's exclusive use.

- A first-aid kit must be on site, and it is recommended that each Practitioner completes first aid training and subsequently repeats that training in accordance with the Health and Safety Executive (HSE) requirements.

- The Practitioner must ensure: health and safety risk assessments of their place of work, fire safety drills and checks, and electrical equipment checks are completed annually by appropriately qualified and approved persons and certificated accordingly.

- Access for disabled persons should be provided at the premises.

- Anyone under the age of 16 must be accompanied by their parent or guardian who must also take full responsibility for signing the consent form prior to any treatment commencing.

- Practitioners must retain (and display) at their place of work a copy of qualification certificates and Code of Ethics.

- Practitioners must be conversant with the legislation that informs the operation of a practice and conduct their business and the maintenance of all the necessary records (including storage) accordingly.

Suggested Framework for Entry Requirements to Colon Hydrotherapy Training Courses

The selection process is invariably based around an interview. The interview provides the best vehicle for ascertaining someone's relevant experience, qualifications, personal qualities, characteristics, as well as their **personal assets.**

The interview will also show if the prospective student is able to express themselves clearly and whether they can articulate their views in a non-dogmatic way which is likely to imply openness to different views and perceptions. **Applicants need:**

- To have been trained in allopathic/conventional medicine, or be graduates of a recognized complementary medicine course and be able to evidence the study of anatomy and physiology at an in-depth level.

- To be able to evidence the equivalent of two years, practice experience, and during that time show evidence of a commitment to CPD.

- To be able to evidence (as appropriate) professional indemnity insurance cover was held during previous practice.

- To have experienced colon hydrotherapy and agree to receive treatments during training.

- To be able to produce copies of certificates of qualifications.

- Complete and return the application form (and curriculum vitae if applicants so choose) and produce two references in support of their application.

- Send with the return of the application form a recent passport-type photograph.

The process of selection focuses upon choosing students with not only the right attributes but also the ability to fully satisfy the above requirements.

Guide to Course Design

The contents of this manual and reference book **reflect the core aspects** of an appropriately designed training course in colon hydrotherapy. Such a course needs to be show flexibility, and best practice standards must be evidenced and discussed throughout the course. The course design must allow for balance between **theoretical and practical** work, and allow time for reflection, and acquisition of skills and knowledge.

The chosen training course is likely to run over approximately 100 hours, including time for examination and viva voce. Forty hours home-study is also recommended. In addition to the student's self-directed home-study, the completion of set assignments and a short dissertation of an associated area of study within the field of complementary medicine is suggested. A course based upon a modular approach to learning, thus providing, as noted, flexibility in teaching, course design, timetabling, and development, is a proven approach to higher education. By the end of the initial modules, the student should be fully aware of many of the issues surrounding colon hydrotherapy, will have received and given colon hydrotherapy treatments, and will be seeing colon hydrotherapy treatment in a wider context of associated treatment regimes. By the end of the subsequent modules and graduation it is expected that the student will have sufficient competence necessary to commence practice as a Registered Colon Hydrotherapist.

As part of the assessment of applied skills 10 case studies (involving two follow-up treatments each) are suggested and evaluation by an external examiner is recommended. Upon satisfactory completion of all aspects of the course students will then, correctly, receive their Diploma.

An essential pre-course reading list, and recommended reference book list, is detailed near the end of this book. Such a list will vary from course to course, as will aspects of course design and emphasis. The foregoing is a guide only.

The Suggested Elements of Training and Learning

Inspiring students to use their potential for maximum **self-realization and personal achievement** is clearly the most important task facing any training programme co-ordinator. Issues like 'I must be competent', 'I must be in control', 'I must be perfect' are some of the beliefs that get in the way of adult learning. It is the course design and the skill of the tutors that will assist students in developing their own personal adequacy, as well as academic and practical competence.

To achieve such goals, learning must take place in an environment that is **emotionally safe and intellectually challenging.** The student is reacting, in part, to that which is being taught, and also the actual learning environment. It is these factors that influence the motivation to learn, and as a consequence, the acquisition of knowledge and new skills.

Hence, a range of teaching materials and approaches are necessary. These will include: lectures, seminars, experiential learning, practical application of skills, clinical practice, and reading lists, and reference material. The organization of the course ensures an appropriate balance between the theoretical and practical aspects of the training programme.

The class will usually comprise no more than four to six students. Clearly, learning in a group has a social quality about it, which can be utilized for discussion of specific teaching points, the sharing of experience, testing of opinions and theories, and sharing of thoughts and feelings. (To a large extent helping equals the sharing of experience so, in one sense, we cannot learn or help unless we attempt to share our experience, and give and receive feedback.)

It is for such reasons that group learning is so often adopted for training in the helping professions. Learning, awareness, and insight are emotional events and as such run contrary to the popular belief that the intellect is the principal avenue of learning. It is the relationship by the student to what is being taught that is critical.

We intuitively know that direct experience is the best teacher and group learning provides the ideal setting to gain direct experience and acquire the necessary skills to become a skilled and able colon hydrotherapist.

It is the combination of teaching approaches made possible within the group, and the chance to share, which actually creates the most meaningful and effective learning opportunities. Group learning also encourages self-evaluation and monitoring of personal progress, which is especially important for the student. Furthermore, such awareness is an essential part of being a good Practitioner.

Emotions and Feelings

Emotions and feelings **are an integral part of the total personality** and, therefore, are of critical concern in **the helping relationship**. A broad range of conditions and circumstances arouse emotion and 'equally' a broad range of emotions and feelings are 'stirred up' and will vary in intensity.

Emotions affect the body and are manifested in symptoms such as increased heartbeat, diarrhoea, constipation, skin problems, thrush, and cystitis. In the workplace and no doubt in our homes we encounter temper, jealousy, despondency, as well as laughter. The range of emotional behaviour for which each is capable is considerable, and will vary from person to person.

Some people have, as a learned response to life, 'preferred' feelings, for example, feeling depressed or ill. As such, individuals define themselves in this way and as a consequence body-energy, their life-force, is immediately and adversely affected.

The more self-aware person leads a richer emotional life, understands and appreciates his or her emotions and feelings for what they are. They will utilize and integrate them with their own wellbeing and the welfare of others in mind. They are able to channel their emotions and the energy these generate into constructive behaviours and concern for their physical and emotional wellbeing in the knowledge of their inter-relatedness. In addition to the obvious physical benefits of colon hydrotherapy Patients will 'feel' better emotionally.

This will demand of the **skilled Practitioner** the ability to address the Patient's life-style and the consequences for health; diet-related matters; allergies and food sensitivities; and the role of supplements and so on.

So, it is clear that in addition to diet one of the other major influences on the bowel is emotional stress. This may begin to explain why more people are admitted to hospital with gastrointestinal complaints than any other malady.

We know that emotional strain affects the body.

Think of that nervous tummy before an interview! Nervous tension causes contractions in all the orifices of the body. When we learn to let go of stress, tension, and negative thoughts, we relax. If the anus is not relaxed at the time of elimination it will be difficult to rid the body of toxins. Remember, autointoxication is the result of intestinal toxaemia. Autointoxication happens when the body absorbs too much of its own toxic waste.

Taking care of oneself involves the integration of experience into a coherent and personally satisfying learning and growing process.

We know that **psychosomatic (mind/body) disorders** are partly attributed to the emotional state of the individual. The most obvious difference among Patients is the part of the body affected. The reason why one particular organ or part of the body suffers is unknown. Psychosomatic disorders are real diseases involving damage to the body. The fact that these are caused by emotional factors does not make the affliction imaginary. People can just as readily die from psychosomatic disorders (asthma/ulcers) as from infection or physical injury. Parts of the body affected include:

- The skin: for example, inflammation, dryness, itching, and eczema.

- Respiration: for example, asthma, sighing, hiccoughs, and breathing rapidly.

- Alimentary canal: for example, ulcers, acidity, heartburn, constipation, and diarrhoea.

- Genito-urinary system: for example, disturbances in menstruation and urination, urinary frequency, and impotence.

- Muscular skeletal system: for example, backache, cramps, and tension headaches.

33

In addition to the above, many other diseases are viewed by some as being partly caused by emotional and psychological factors, for example, multiple sclerosis, pneumonia, cancer, and the common cold.

Clearly, the emotional state of the Patient is now recognized as playing a critical role in illness and its treatment. Put at its most simple – "I feel happy I am well", "I feel unhappy I am sick".

All functioning and all diseases are both mental and physical as both of these aspects of our body and life are going on continuously. As such this emphasizes a **naturopathic** and 'holistic' approach to treatment especially as it strongly suggests we are considering and treating a monistic system rather than a dualistic one. It is for the biologically and physiologically orientated theorists to explain why some people develop given symptoms and what determines the particular symptom or disorder!?

It is stated in the ancient acupuncture texts that if the mind is at peace the body will not be susceptible to disease, even infections. In Chinese Medicine, behaviour is actually classified according to five primary emotional and behavioural tendencies. These are tendencies to have: outbursts of rage and anger; excessive joy or emotion; inappropriate reflection and worry; sadness and withdrawal; and fear.

By acting selectively on a meridian and on an organ, each of these tendencies are said to disorganize the bodily systems in very specific ways. For example, anger in excess harms the liver and gallbladder; fear affects the bowel and associated organs; joy affects the heart; the spleen is affected by reflection; and the lungs are affected by sadness. (Requena Y, 1989).

The benefits of understanding our own psychology, strengths, and weaknesses has been emphasized since Socrates made his now-accepted directive **'Know Thyself'**. Our individual behaviours are often in a direct rapport with our biological activities. Other times we subject ourselves to biological variations caused by stress, such as the abuse of stimulants and so on. To know our self better permits and enables us to become more responsible in all our choices.

It is worth noting here, that one of Sigmund Freud's major discoveries was that **psychosomatic/psychological illness is the fear of knowledge of oneself**, of one's emotions, impulses, memories, and the potentialities of one's life as a whole.

Many in fact live, as the Danish philosopher Soren Kierkegaard put it, by 'tranquillizing themselves with the trivial'. By facing up to the often unpleasant and difficult aspects of our life, and all its symptoms, 'destroys the lie', and becomes both health enhancing and liberating.

Part of the case-taking role means that the colon hydrotherapist acts as a sounding board and sometimes a 'vessel' for the Patient's emotions. Feelings shared by others can arouse feelings in us. **Two factors will determine how effective the therapist will be:**

- Their own strength in terms of their own self-awareness and knowledge of the source and meaning of their own feelings.

- The degree of emotional pressure the 'contents' of the feelings, be they the ones expressed by the Patient, or the ones held by the Therapist.

Again, one is reminded of the requirement of the Practitioner to be active around their CPD and self-understanding.

Also rudimentary to best practice, but so often forgotten, is for the therapist to **avoid the desire to give advice to the Patient.** For example, "If I was you, I wouldn't worry about what you are worrying about" or, "The answer to your problem is my belief system" or, "You must do as I say". Such interventions are always inappropriate as giving advice negates the Patient's own capacity to think, choose, and resolve, to their own satisfaction, their own issues. Obviously, the Patient comes for advice regarding symptom-based concerns. To respond appropriately requires insight, knowledge, and experience. What are not warranted are unrelated, unhelpful, and potentially very damaging simplistic statements, which in reality, reflect the Practitioner's agenda, and therefore, has little to do with the needs of the Patient.

Discussion of symptoms, and their possible causes, must be approached from the principle of **enabling or empowering** the Patient to find their own 'helper within themselves', as well as taking responsibility for the implementation of any resulting treatment regime.

The Philosophy Informing Helping and Issues for Practice

The following philosophy fully **takes into full account the fact that thinking, feeling, and behavioural problems behind disease and dysfunction are usually learned and become habitual.** Therefore, these can be 'unlearned' or replaced with more satisfying and health-enhancing choices. The majority of Patient's seeking colon hydrotherapy are not seriously ill but are, in the main, individuals seeking treatment for specific symptoms, comfort, guidance in the process of 'growing', change in personal circumstances, **coping, and living.**

Change is often conceived of pain and turmoil, and arises not only from health-related factors, but wider factors like the wish to change old patterns of behaving, unhealthy habits, diet, and a general wish to take greater care of oneself. **The philosophy informing the helping professions places the Patient, and their responsibility, at the centre of the process:**

- That people are capable and therefore able to participate, and be responsible for, their own change programme.

- That on some level, people know what they need to do in order to resolve personal difficulties, conflicts, and health issues.

- That all the transactions (verbal, non-verbal, and physical) between the Patient and Practitioner are a part of the helping process.

- That inappropriate behaviour is confronted within the 'here and now' (to bring into the Patient's awareness).

- That confrontation is equal to caring and being passive (doing or saying nothing) is equal to not caring. (Schiff J, 1975).

Helping is facilitated by the Practitioner developing a climate in which the Patient feels relaxed, is able to be direct and open, and feels safe.

The success of the process depends upon the performance of the Practitioner. How well they use their intuition, and training, and how successfully they are able to relate to the Patient. **Competence** is fundamental to any consideration of **effectiveness.** As noted elsewhere in this book observing the Codes of Ethics, Codes of Practice, and the Philosophy Informing Helping is absolute, also:

- Informing the Patient of the methods and principles to be adopted as well as the expected duration of sessions and the fee (if any) to be charged.

- Exploring with the Patient their expectations of the visit and/or, treatment session.

- Confirming with the Patient whether or not they are currently involved in any other treatment with another Practitioner and gaining the Patient's permission to discuss with them any such interventions, and/or permission, if considered necessary, for the Colon Hyrotherapist Practitioner to confer with the other Practitioner/s, other Professional/s.

- The Practitioner is taking account of their own competence, monitoring their own competence, and suggesting alternative referrals as appropriate.

- Terminating helping when the Practitioner is satisfied that the Patient has received the help sought, or when it is apparent that the help being provided is no longer of benefit.

- Approaching helping from a position of humility with the understanding that each of us has needs, both the Practitioner and the Patient, and that in different circumstances or situation, the roles could be reversed.

Being aware of the fact that the Patient has strengths and abilities and that all of us experience many of the same things as joy, sadness, aches, and pains! Facing an issue, confronting a problem or symptom, implies having at least some information about the 'symptom' otherwise it would obviously be outside of the Patient's awareness. Therefore, the Practitioner aims to **enhance** the Patient's **understanding** of the symptom/s through further clarification of the problem area and further investigation is likely to include breaking the symptom/s down into more manageable parts prior to the formulation of any treatment plan.

Considering a Treatment Plan

One of the faults in all forms of problem-solving is that we are prone to decide on a remedy before the symptoms and underlying causes have been sufficiently explored or understood. Always, and without exception, the Patient is invited to complete a **Treatment Consent Form,** (See Table 10). This is absolutely necessary in order to empower the Patient by underlining their decision to seek treatment, and if they wished to conclude treatment, and placing that decision within their control. Moreover, it is important from the outset to quietly establish boundaries by explaining to the Patient the counter indications and limits to colon hydrotherapy and by doing so is clearly in the best interests of the Patient.

The colon hydrotherapist is trained to diagnose imbalances and breakdowns within the body's own self-healing abilities. In administering a colon hydrotherapy the therapist will also be educating the Patient to become empowered and in charge of their own health.

A meaningful treatment plan depends upon a thorough understanding and diagnosis of the Patient by considering aspects of their lifestyle, thinking, diet, feelings, bowel movements, exercise, rest, sleep, possible causes, and so on.

By addressing the relevant questions the Practitioner and the Patient will be able to be more precise about the nature and likely causes of the symptom/s. This in turn will provide a deeper understanding of any associated issues influencing the symptoms, thus being essential for both meaningful diagnosis, and any course of treatment.

The sum of this process, including understanding and clarifying information provided by the Patient in the **case taking form**, will help confirm if further analysis and investigation is required. For example, a medical examination may be indicated. Together the Practitioner and Patient will be able to agree on the best way forward. (See Consultation Form, Table 11).

Remember, **for a treatment plan to be effective in its implementation it has to be 'owned' by the Patient.** Practitioner skill and knowledge will ensure in-depth and critical analysis, in order to 'prevent' the Patient from accepting and being satisfied with less than the appropriate treatments or remedies. The Practitioner should now know:

- What symptom/s (underlying cause/s) have (hopefully) been identified.
- Will have, in concrete terms, a symptom picture.
- Know what is distinctive about the symptom/s (for example, worse when cold, worse after certain foods.
- Know where the symptom is and where it is not.
- Will know if symptoms have changed during the time they occurred, for example, becoming worse, or the ache has moved.
- Know what the Patient intends to do and what they cannot do now.
- Know what changes the Patient wishes to make, for example, more exercise, improved diet.
- Be clear about the Patient's priorities and their ability to choose appropriate goals.
- The Patient will be clear about the implications of the chosen treatment goals, for example, daily commitments, and timings for supplements.
- Know whether the Patient has support or the resources to proceed satisfactorily with the plan.
- Whether they will need to involve others (in their immediate family/relationships) or require their co-operation (for example, concerning a major change in diet).
- Time scales for treatment regime, and follow-up treatment.

41

- What other information may be available to improve understanding or options and what alternative treatments may be useful.

The Patient will hopefully know the answer to four questions:

- What am I to do?

- When am I to do it?

- How am I going to do it?

- Why am I doing it?

Also remember, **keep an accurate record of symptoms and discussion**, for it is often surprising how, as a course of treatment progresses, Patients forget about difficulties that were once of immediate concern and have now, due to successful intervention, ceased to be so. For example, I recall asking a Patient for an update on whether there had been improvement regarding the headaches which six months previously had been one of several symptoms discussed. Being no longer affected in this way the Patient had forgotten that headaches had once been a real problem. **Without good records any meaningful evaluation of progress becomes impossible.**

Reviewing a Treatment Plan

This stage is the examination of the success or otherwise of the recommended treatment, how well it has been followed, and its appropriateness. It needs to be borne in mind that **there is an interrelationship between every aspect of the helping process. From actually meeting with the Patient, taking the case, diagnosis, developing the treatment plan, to the review of that plan post-implementation.** These elements are best seen as not being separate elements in themselves, but as part of a whole.

The Practitioner is now **seeking clarity** from the Patient as follows:

- Has there been any improvement?

- To what extent has the plan been effective?

- Were some parts more successful than others?

- What parts of the plan require further consideration and adjustment?

- What parts, if any, require further consideration, examination, and definition?

- To what extent does the Patient remain committed to and motivated by the plan?

- Are there alternative solutions?

- Have elements of the plan been overlooked, neglected, or only partially adhered to?

- How does the Patient now think and feel about the treatment and its relationship to symptoms?

- How do significant others now think and feel about the treatment plan?

- Finally, is it still the 'right' plan?

Throughout all the elements of the process the Practitioner is **facilitating the Patient** to identify the symptoms, checking for specific details (for example, nature of the pain, type of pain), exploring or reconciling apparent contradictions and placing the symptoms (or new symptoms) in the context of the Patient's life and lifestyle.

The chosen treatment plan is sometimes ineffective not because it is poorly implemented but because it, or aspects of it, are inappropriate. The treatment plan may be based upon an adequate understanding of the symptoms but an inadequate choice of options to their treatment. For example, colon hydrotherapy will certainly improve health but aches in the body due to an overburdened liver may require treatment specific to the liver.

Moreover, every treatment plan incorporates within it a theory of what is the problem and cause. If the treatment fails it may be that the theory is at fault, rather than the treatment plan or its execution.

Other learned habits may also impede effective treatment, including poor motivation. Such will be explored during the review of progress. Moreover, the Patient may find one aspect of the plan unacceptable or difficult to achieve, which may destroy the whole plan.

If the treatment plan is based upon a faulty assessment or inadequate knowledge and experience, the chances of error are clearly increased. Hence, the need for the Practitioner to establish ongoing monitoring and analysis of the Patient's progress and establish regular liaison, supervision, and **consultation** with experienced and competent colleagues.

The Practitioner can:

- Look at and evaluate the entire process with Patients.
- Select points in the process, for example the case-taking stage, and ask 'am I satisfied with my performance and my skills'?
- Examine the quality of their interaction with the Patient, any specific difficulties, mistakes, and so on.

- Review their progress by asking for feedback.
- Take case studies to your professional practice supervisor.

Self-evaluation by the Practitioner is an integral aspect of the total helping process. Such ongoing evaluation provides the information upon which the Practitioner's further development and training can be planned and guided.

Often overlooked, because the issues may be very sensitive, is the question of the **termination of treatment.** In certain cases the treatment may reach a point of diminishing returns for the Patient and the Practitioner, for example, when the time and expense begin to outweigh the benefits the Patient is receiving. We are not here discussing Patients who are receiving, as part of an active and overall treatment plan, ongoing maintenance support and treatment, but of those cases where there is a real sense that the degree of benefit and progress being achieved fails to justify continuation.

Clearly, the final **decision about conclusion** will involve the Practitioner and the Patient. The Practitioner's responsibility is to provide feedback which is empathic, nurturing, and enabling regarding their perception of how the Patient is progressing, especially with regard to the agreed Treatment Plan and goals. It may be the time to consider other possible modalities, and possible referral to other Practitioners. The Practitioner must be clear and honest in the knowledge that there will always be Patient's for whom, and for various reasons, are to work with, or to continue to work with, and **this must be acknowledged.**

The Principles of Natural Therapeutics

Colon hydrotherapy is a naturopathic treatment. It works naturally with the body's healing power and self-correcting mechanisms. The colon hydrotherapist works in accordance with the following **naturopathic principles:**

- The body possesses an innate ability to heal itself, therefore the therapist works with body's healing power, uses treatments which also do the same, and avoids treatments that may work against these natural mechanisms.

- Deviation from the natural biological laws, and as a consequence a state of lost bodily equilibrium, results in **disease**. Hence, there is always an underlying cause to disease, be it physical, psychological, or emotional (called by naturopaths the **Triad of Health**) which recognizes the natural relationship, connection, and interaction between these aspects of our bodily function and our life. In other words, treating the whole person. Health is therefore more than the **absence of disease,** it is also a state of physical, psychological, and emotional wellbeing.

- Dysfunction in one area invariably leads to dysfunction else-where. **Health and disease** therefore represent a continuum that ranges from the absolute optimum of bodily performance and wellbeing to the extreme of degeneration, close to death.

- So, because health and disease are a process, not literally states or conditions, they must be seen as relative terms that are constantly altering in one direction or the other. Health and disease are concepts that describe function or performance of the cell, organ, or bodily systems. Health is normal function, disease is abnormal function.

Health reflects a dynamic quality where the **internal** performance of the bodily environment is conducive to its survival (although it seems genetic and congenital factors will impose limitations). With disease, the internal environment is not conducive to survival, there has been a disturbance or challenge to balance (homoeostasis), and the 'life-force' is endeavouring to influence physiological action, defend against cause, and utilize repair and immunity, in order to restore a more conducive environment. When this fails disease is manifested. Therefore, degeneration is the result of persistent physiological threats occurring in the body that remain ignored (often outside of our awareness) and remain unremoved.

Colon hydrotherapy will not cure on its own, but can provide the cleansed environment necessary for a better future!

The recognition of the existence of a vital curative force within the body (often referred to as the vital force or life force) means that treatment is aimed at **improving curative energy** by using various physical and biological stimuli to activate and strengthen bodily equilibrium (homoeostasis). This means using agents and techniques found naturally. For example, water, herbs, adjustment of diet, exercise, and rest. Also adjustment and changes to our relationship to environmental (pollutants) and social factors. Note: the increasing burden on the body of **iatrogenic** disease, which is disease resulting from medical treatments, and their side effects.

Adherence to the laws of natural living will enhance the body's capacity to cure and by removing toxic substances and situations from our lifestyle, works to prevent the onset of disease/further disease. Prevention is better than cure!

The traditional treatments of acupressure and reflexology **claim** to utilize energy lines or meridians, and reflex points, to treat both symptoms and causes. (See Figure 7 Pressure Points). Disturbance to the body's **'vibrational' potential** is due to: lowered vitality, abnormal composition of blood and lymph, and the accumulation of morbid materials and poisons. (Lindlahr H, 1975).

The human organism is, therefore, a dynamic, automatically adjusting structure. Its stability is provided by the continuous operation of different physiological systems, thus changing the physical properties of biological tissues, temperature, magnetic permeability, and electrical impedance. (Makerenko & Pirotti, 2001).

Although most worthy of further scientific study and explanation, let us acknowledge the efforts of Practitioners from earlier times whose treatments goals spoke of such factors as: achieving balance between bodily energies, altering bodily rhythms, affecting energy lines, altering vibrations, moving of energies, making use of pressure points, using the breath to help to create equilibrium, meditation, relaxation, massage, working with Chi, awareness of the Chakras; all linking the body and mind in order to create balance, reduce stress, and create inner harmony.

It is clear that colon hydrotherapy will assist in **improving** and balancing **elimination.** Through detoxification of the body, **digestion** will be improved as **absorption and excretion** become appropriately balanced. Dietary adjustment will also improve, for example, **blood-sugar levels** and help **balance the hormonal system,** for example, the adrenal and thyroid glands.

The process of cure is the re-adjustment of the human organism from abnormal to normal conditions and functioning. No matter what the final symptoms or underlying pathology the same **causative sequence of disease** arising in five phases are as follows: (Issels J, 1975).

- **Causal factors,** for example, constitutional, genetic, structural, emotional, and nutritional, will lead to such conditions as abnormal intestinal flora/balance. (Note: the **healthy bowel has around 85% friendly lactobacillus bacteria and around 15% unfriendly gas producing, *Bacillus coli*).**

- **Secondary damage,** for example, to cells, liver, intestines, and excretory system leading to toxicity.

- **Disease milieu**, leading to lowered resistance and immunity, metabolic disturbance.

- **Susceptibility to infection,** pathological damage, the development of disease.

- **Disease symptoms,** for example, local inflammation, pain, necrosis (the death of some or all the cells in an organ or tissue), cysts, tumours, fever, fatigue, blood dyscrasia (abnormal state of the body or part of the body), anxiety, and depression.

As the result of evidence from his own investigations, analysis, and findings the German homoeopath Constantine Hering (who emigrated to America in the 1830s), observed that healing also occurs in a consistent pattern. He described this pattern in the form of three basic laws that homoeopaths can use to see that healing is occurring. This pattern is used by acupuncturists, herbalist, and other healing disciplines.

According to Hering, the **first law of cure** is that healing progresses from the deepest part of the organism. Therefore, it develops from the mental and emotional levels and from the vital organs outward, to the external parts of organism (our body) such as the skin and extremities (hands, feet). This reflects the body's attempts to externalize disease, to dislodge it from the more serious internal levels/organs to the more 'superficial' external levels. Thus, someone with asthma may develop an external skin rash as part of the curative process.

The **second law** of cure states that as healing progresses symptoms appear and disappear in reverse order to their original appearance. The last symptoms to appear will be the first to go.

Hering's **third law** states that healing progresses from the upper parts of the body to the lower parts of the body. For example, a person is considered to be improving when pains that were once in their shoulders have now moved to their hips. As healing progresses, moving outwards and downwards from the deepest and higher parts of the body respectively, it is possible that the Patient may experience individual symptoms becoming worse (known as a healing crisis) than they were before treatment was sought.

If the Patient is truly healing they will feel stronger and somewhat better despite the aggravation, which before long will pass and leave the Patient healthier at all levels.

A healing crisis is the opposite of a disease yet in many ways feels the same. Symptoms are often similar although it is essential to make the distinction between the symptoms of disease and those of the healing and treatment process. The healing crisis usually occurs after a period of increased wellbeing and may last for several days. Each healing crises releases problems from the past, do not attempt to stop it! This may confuse the Patient when the discomfort they feel is an indication of the body working to heal itself, from the inside out.

The healing crisis can activate the location of chronic settlements and toxins that create a weakness in the body. When old waste matter is disturbed it returns to the bloodstream and the process of elimination commences. It may be unpleasant to experience but necessary for healing to take place. As we know, one of the fastest and effective methods to promote healing is detoxification through colon hydrotherapy.

Our health depends upon many factors. Colon hydrotherapists pay particular attention to toxaemia theories. These are based upon the belief that waste products of metabolism plus chemical toxins from food, (including free radicals), drugs, and the environment, accumulate in the tissues causing cellular damage. This damage then obstructs the vital functions of the cells, including the accumulation of 'morbid matter'.

In all parts of the gastrointestinal tract there are glandular cells that secrete toxins. A large part of the faeces consists of such secretions.

There is increasing evidence to suggest that the rate of transit time is directly related to degenerative diseases. The need for fresh, natural foods with plenty of roughage is essential for healthy intestinal function, including the mechanical function of elimination and the development of beneficial intestinal flora. (See Figure 2, Food Transit Times).

Retained faeces will lead to a state of **'dysbacteria'** which is an abnormal mix of bacteria, which is considered to be a cause of cancer and other degenerative diseases. (Turner R N, 2000).

Moreover, changes in the permeability of the intestinal walls may lead to **autointoxication** and grossly damage the intestinal flora, which are also destroyed by antibiotics, steroids, and non-steroidal anti-inflammatory drugs. Where possible, let us utilize simple treatments before the more complex.

Many of the foregoing guiding principles can be traced back to Hippocrates (460–377BCE). The Hippocratic Oath (believed to have been written by Hippocrates), traditionally taken by physicians to refer to the ethical practice of medicine, was updated by the World Medical Association Declaration of Geneva, Physicians Oath (1948). In the United Kingdom, the General Medical Council provides clear modern guidance in the form of its 'Duties of a Doctor' and 'Good Medical Practice'.

Naturopathy has been described as the Western equivalent to Ayurvedic medicine (from India) and traditional Chinese Medicine, each being a total philosophy of health and life, rather than a 'cure' for specific symptoms and diseases.

The History of Colon Hydrotherapy

Colon hydrotherapy is a very **ancient method** of treatment and healing. The use of enemas was recorded by the Egyptians as early as 1,500BCE, found in the 'Ebers of Papyrus', the earliest-known medical book, although it is known that the Chinese used such methods long before then. Moreover, Ayurvedic medicine included colon cleansing as did Hippocrates in Greece and Galen in Rome. In these earlier times people would use a hollow reed to allow the water to flow into the rectum for cleansing, help maintain health, and avoid disease.

The popularity of colon hydrotherapy reached its apex in the 1920s to 1940s during which time it was used regularly by doctors in surgeries and hospitals. Since then, the use of this valuable health treatment significantly decreased until the resurgence of interest in complementary medicine during the last 10 years or so.

This 'grass-roots' movement towards people taking direct personal responsibility for their healthcare has given momentum to a return to this time-proven method of bowel and health management. The development of sophisticated colon irrigation machines and disposable equipment make this therapy both safe and convenient, adding to its current popularity and understanding of the benefits of maintaining a biologically balanced colon.

The basis of modern hydrotherapy was first discussed in the book, 'Colon Hygiene' by Dr John Harvey Kellogg (1916). Also, by the herbalist Jethro Kloss, in his book 'Back to Eden' (1939), that remains in print. In the 1930s, Dr Bernard Jensen administered thousands of colonics and the testimonials he received, stating the benefits of the treatment, helped at that time to popularize colon hydrotherapy.

Many natural therapists believe that **death begins in the colon** (known as the bowel, or known anatomically as the large intestine). Being the major organ of elimination the colon is susceptible to stagnation and the formation of decay and poisonous deposits.

Therefore, it is essential to keep the colon free from putrefaction otherwise the products of decay spread beyond the colon to other organs causing a sort of autointoxication. Such poisoning may take many different forms. (See Figure 1, The Colon)

For example, in the brain and nervous system, it causes irritability and depression; in the heart, weakness and low energy; in the lungs, breathlessness and halitosis; in the digestive system, bloating and discomfort; in the blood, sallow and spotty skin. The general pace of toxaemia may lead for example, to stomach ulcers, cancers, colitis, insomnia, muscle atrophy, and liver and kidney disease.

Moreover, in a report to the Royal Society of Medicine (1912) 36 poisonous substances were listed as causing, in the smallest quantities, the most profound effects. It would be reasonable to extrapolate from this that given today's use of additives, preservatives, insecticides, the range of chemicals used in household cleaners, stored in the garage, and chemicals used in the production of cosmetics, means that the situation has declined significantly rather than improved!

Many of us experience varying degrees of diarrhoea, constipation, flatulence, and other digestive difficulties. As we have seen, the use of water to cleanse the colon has been practised for centuries. Colon hydrotherapy not **only cleanses the colon, it helps to detoxify the whole body.**

"Colonic irrigation is an undervalued and often forgotten treatment option, which deserves its rightful place among the other treatment modalities." (Kock S M)

"Irrigation of the distal part of the large bowel might be considered as a non-surgical alternative for patients with impaired continence" (Briel J W)

Critics and Controversy

Of course, colon hydrotherapy has its critics and controversy. Some people are critical about colon hydrotherapy washing out beneficial intestinal flora, there is the risk of perforation of the colon, and that there is a risk of contamination. The important fact is that putrefied toxic material is removed, thus creating a positive environment for the assimilation of nutrients and a place where positive bacteria are able to flourish. There is no recorded case of perforation happening. It must be remembered that the water pressure administered is negligible compared with the pressure that can be exerted during normal defecation. Colon hydrotherapy machines incorporate a valve system that prevents soiled water from returning to the water supply. Disposable equipment is used for each Patient and after every treatment.

Colon hydrotherapy practice recognizes that we are all affected by what we each consume. Any toxic by-products will potentially damage the intestinal walls and be absorbed into the blood and lymph fluids, and then ultimately to the tissues and cells. Peristalsis becomes weak, causing a **slower transit of food through the alimentary canal.** This increases fermentation and putrefaction of undigested food, creating gases and toxic waste. Thus, elimination becomes incomplete and faecal waste remains in the colon. Dehydration and stagnation results, creating the conditions in the body called disease!

The Principles of Colon Hydrotherapy

Understanding the principles of hydrotherapy will enable us to appreciate the **significance of the use of water** in colon hydrotherapy.

We know that by drinking plenty of water the contents of the intestines become more fluid thus facilitating elimination. Water also removes poisonous waste from the blood by dissolving poisons whenever it comes into contact with them, thus rendering the blood, tissues, and organs, cleaner. Water is an **excellent solvent** due to the polarity of the water molecule and its tendency to form hydrogen bonds with other molecules.

Note: Ionized water is the product of an electrolytic reaction that takes in an ionized water unit and separates negative ions (alkaline) and positive ions (acid). There is a growing body of evidence to show that drinking alkaline water helps rid the body of acid waste. Such water also alkalizes the body and provides an effective antioxidant. Alkaline water is being recommended when conditions of over- acidity develop, (colds, flu) and for toxic and high acid conditions such as arthritis. (Baroody T, 2005). Acid water (pH -3) can and is being used as a disinfectant and replacement for herbicides and related usage, as bacteria cannot survive that level of acidity.

When we drink pure, fresh water, the body is bathed and purified. A large number of diseases are caused by the obstruction of the various organs by the accumulation of waste material. Warm water applied externally opens the pores to enable elimination, and water taken by mouth will relieve internal obstruction due to it being the most effective solvent we have!

Most of us are also familiar with the value of applying **hot and cold compresses** to the skin in order to achieve a deeper reaction within the body. For example, we apply cold water on bumps in order to reduce swelling; warm/hot water compresses applied to the chest will help to loosen phlegm so it can be more easily coughed up.

Moreover, rapidly drinking several glasses of tepid water will, as required, act as an **emetic** and cause vomiting; drinking plenty of water, as a **diuretic**, will increase the amount of urine produced; a warm bath helps us to relax and sleep more soundly; a hot or cold shower acts as a stimulant; a hot fomentation (poultice) acts as an analgesic thus relieving pain by increasing local circulation, it will also soften skin to allow matter to be expressed; the pulse rate can be reduced by taking a cool bath; the body temperature will decrease by bathing in water below 98°Fahrenheit (approximately 33° centigrade). Life on earth totally depends on water, and given that the human body is two-thirds water it is not surprising that **water is remedially so effective.**

The chemical reactions in all plants and animals that support life take place in a water medium. In short, the chemistry of life is water chemistry.

Water is composed of two gases: hydrogen and oxygen. Both are odourless, colourless, and tasteless, and burn rapidly. Oxygen is the most effective supporter of combustion known, and hydrogen is one of the lightest gases known.

Water requires a greater amount of energy to elevate its temperature a given number of degrees than any other substance. Water also conducts heat by giving its heat to surfaces it comes into contact. It also removes heat when it is at a lower temperature than the surfaces it comes into contact with.

With the exception of air there is no other element in nature that is so important for sustaining life than water.

As noted, the performance of each of the body's vital functions depends upon water. The circulatory system depends upon water. With the aid of water, nutrients enter the blood and are taken to where they are needed for growth, repair, and energy.

There is absolutely no other substance other than water

able to pass through the most delicate of capillaries without friction, or pass through membranes without openings. Water is continuously passing out of the body through the skin, lungs, kidneys, and intestines. The average person eliminates up to three litres of water in 24 hours and an equal amount must be provided to preserve the fluidity of the blood. Therefore, diet is directly related to the amount of water demanded by the body. The consumption of animal products, salt, and spices requires considerably more water to dissolve and cleanse the system. People who eat mostly fruit, vegetables, and grains require less water as many fruits and vegetables are more than half water.

As noted, water is the basis of the **body fluids, blood plasma, lymph, and the tissue fluids.** Water acts as a solvent for the important salts of sodium, potassium, and other minerals necessary for metabolism. There is a very important balance between salt and water intake and output which in health, is maintained at a steady level, but which may be seriously upset in disease. Water is, therefore, required for effective elimination. Urine and sweat both consist of 90% water. Water is also excreted by the lungs as vapour, and by the bowels in faeces.

In health there is a constant balance between the intracellular fluid (occurring inside the cell), and the extracellular fluid (occurring outside the cell). This is maintained largely by the process of **osmotic pressure.** When salts are dissolved in water their minute molecules exert pressure on the walls of the structure containing the solution. The walls of the cells and capillaries are membranes through which water and molecules can pass.

The pressure exerted by the molecules is called osmotic pressure and the degree of pressure is dependent on the number of molecules present.

Water, salts, and waste products are constantly passing backwards and forwards between the plasma, tissue fluids, and cells. At the same time, the osmotic pressures of all three are kept constant and maintained by water passing from the weaker tissue placing fluid into the cells until their osmotic pressures are equal (isotonic). If there is water deficiency in the body, plasma and tissue fluids become more concentrated (hypertonic) and water will be extracted from the cells, which then become dehydrated. On the other hand, if there is too much salt in the body water is retained and not excreted by the kidneys. Such accumulation leads to oedema (swelling caused by excessive accumulation of fluid in the body tissues, also known as dropsy).

There may also be serious loss of fluid in cases of severe vomiting, excessive sweating, and diarrhoea, again leading to the condition of dehydration.

Let us not forget that the **lymph system is part of the circulatory system** and a major organ of the immune system. One of its main functions is to transport nutrients to the cells and to remove waste. Waste is taken via the lacteals (lymphatic vessels that extend into the villi of the small intestine) that empty waste into the small intestine (and absorb digested fats). The waste then passes into the colon for elimination. When the intestinal walls are impacted the lymph system retains the waste. If accompanied by dehydration the stage is set for impaired immunity, and constipation! (See The Five Systems of Elimination section).

In colon hydrotherapy, water is used to provide a treatment for the elimination of waste and cleansing of the colon. The process also helps to restore one of the colon's main functions that is the absorption of large amounts of water and electrolytes, groups of atoms that produce electricity, from the undigested food passed on from the small intestine and to produce, at intervals, strong peristaltic movements which move the dehydrated contents, the faeces, towards the rectum for elimination.

The colon hydrotherapy treatment involves the use of warm, filtered water, at low pressure (approximately 0.90Kg per 6.45cm^2; 2lb per square inch), being introduced into the Patient's colon. This happens while the Patient is lying comfortably on a treatment couch. The warm, filtered water flows through a shaped tube known as a speculum that is placed into the anus, about 50mm, and remains in place throughout the treatment. Two tubes are connected to the external part of the speculum. A smaller diameter tube (around 1.3cm) is used to pass the water into the Patient. A larger diameter tube is used to allow for the removal of the colon contents, which are passed via a water trap and anti-siphon valve into the soil pipe. The amount of water circulated through the colon during a single treatment could be around 50 litres.

The **initial examination** of the Patient's **abdomen** requires **a gentle** 'massage'. This is to ascertain the volume of any wind that may be present, the presence of impacted faeces, and possible blockages. By gently feeling the Patient's abdomen the Practitioner will also be able to check for areas of sensitivity and the Patient's level of relaxation while being touched. This initial examination helps prepare the Patient for the more rigorous 'massage' during the colon hydrotherapy treatment.

While receiving the treatment the Patient's **abdomen is massaged** more firmly and deeply. The direction should be across the colon, right to left, in a half-circular motion, in order to help loosen any impacted faecal material now being softened, and sluiced by water. It is also usual to commence from the ileocaecal valve and finish to the left of the bladder. Palpation of the liver and spleen, when appropriate, under the ribcage is also useful in achieving a positive outcome for the Patient.

Time needs to be spent 'massaging' the abdomen in places where resistance is felt. Progress is being made when the entire colon beneath the ribcage softens and good elimination is observed. At all times the Practitioner must aim to keep the Patient relaxed, work deeply as appropriate, but always mindful of both the Patient's 'comfort' and complete awareness of what is happening beneath the fingers.

The Practitioner needs to always be alert to any discomforts the Patient may be feeling, during or after treatment. Nausea may indicate that the liver or gallbladder is congested. A hot flush, or shivering cold, may suggest that the kidneys or hormones are deficient. Blushing may indicate hypertension. Energy levels diminishing rapidly may indicate the spleen, or pancreas, (hypoglycaemia, diabetes).

The **abdominal muscles** are a group of six muscles that extend from various places on the pelvis. They provide movement and support to the trunk and they also assist in the process of breathing. The deeper the muscle is located, that is the closer to the spine, the more powerful effect it will have for creating and maintaining a healthy spine posture. From deep to superficial the abdominal muscles are:

Transverse abdominal, this muscle cannot be touched from the outside of the body, it wraps around the torso creating an effect similar to a back-support belt.

The internal oblique muscles are a pair of muscles situated each side of the torso which are involved in rotation and lateral flexion of the spine.

The external oblique muscles, are another pair of muscles that are located on either side of the torso. They are more superficial and are also involved in rotation and flexion of the spine.

The rectus abdominus, is the most superficial but still affects posture, just not as much as the deeper oblique and transverse muscles. The rectus abdominus muscle is responsible for the 'six-pack' abdominal look in some very fit people.

As the muscles work in groups the abdominal muscles are called spinal flexors. Their main job is to bend the spine forward. The back muscles counterbalance the action of the abdominal muscles and are called spinal **extensors**. In other words, when one set of muscles shortens the other set of muscles stretch, and viceversa. The abdominal muscles participate in the breathing process, especially during exhalation, when they help force air out of the lungs by depressing the thorax.

So, the gentle massaging of the abdomen is an essential aspect of colon hydrotherapy in aiding the movement and effect of the water, and as such, water is enabled to eventually progress through the entire length of the colon. This irrigation of the colon eliminates waste (sometimes built up over many years), mucous, morbid matter, parasites, toxins, and gas.

The colon effectively regains its functions and full peristaltic movement is restored. Regular and complete elimination is encouraged, vital energy levels within the body return, and with a review of diet and lifestyle wellbeing is established.

For optimum health the colon must be functioning normally. As water stimulates the colon mucosa and muscles there is little danger of colon hydrotherapy treatment making the colon lazy, in fact it is the opposite that is the case.

A Synopsis of the Key Issues Concerning New Patients

The **purpose of colon hydrotherapy is the removal of toxic waste material** including: impacted faeces, accumulated mucous, parasites, worms, and unfriendly bacteria. The gentle filling of and emptying of water into and from the colon improves muscular contraction (peristalsis) and elimination. **This treatment process helps to restore the colon to health and consequently, enables it to perform all of its functions more efficiently.**

In a single treatment session approximately **50l of water** will be used to gently flush the colon and through the use of stomach massage and the use of pressure points the therapist will facilitate the elimination of the toxic waste.

The colon muscles contract and relax expelling liquid, gas, and waste, into the rectum creating a feeling of the need to empty, which as the Patient relaxes will follow as normal. The Therapist will appreciate the sensitivity of the procedure and will help the Patient to feel at ease. After the gentle insertion of the speculum into the rectum and the introduction of warm filtered water, plastic tubing simply carries the waste away.

Colon hydrotherapy treatments are pleasant, painless, and discreet. If painful experiences happen they usually result from the Patient being tense and resistant to the treatment. The skilled therapist will minimize discomfort by putting the Patient at ease. There is intrinsically no danger in colon hydrotherapy and is, essentially, a natural process. Moreover, the Patient's modesty is preserved and maintained at all times. During the treatment itself, the Patient will be fully covered and all personal and medical details will be treated with total confidentiality.

Patients suffering from constipation benefit from increasing fluid intake and fibre in advance of treatment. Treatments are assisted if the Patient has evacuated the bowel prior to the treatment session.

It is best for the Patient to arrive for their treatment five minutes before their appointment to allow for time to relax and, if necessary, to use the toilet. There is no danger of bowel perforation and the equipment used in each treatment is sterilized and disposed of after use. The clinic is disinfected using hospital-approved disinfectant.

The Patient is advised to eat or drink only lightly in the two hours preceding a colonic. After the colonic, the Patient is likely to feel a sense of wellbeing. A cup of refreshing mint tea is recommended before continuing their day. The colonic may stimulate, in the next few hours, several bowel movements, however these will not be sudden, uncontrollable, or painful, but rather the colon performing its function by **eliminating waste efficiently.**

Sometimes, when the colon is weak or sluggish there may be no bowel movement for several days. This is likely to be an indication that further treatments are necessary to strengthen and heal the colon so that other additional treatments and changes in diet and lifestyle are able to produce beneficial effects.

Occasionally, and usually due to the extra water introduced to the colon, diarrhoea or loose bowels may be experienced. If this should occur it is usually of short duration.

The **number of treatments** required will vary from Patient to Patient and be dependent upon the treatment goals. For example, a course of treatments in order to improve the health of the colon and to address other various symptoms may require a series of treatments over a year or more; or, just one initial treatment followed by monthly maintenance treatments. The therapist will plan with the Patient suggested requirements, the recommended number of treatments, and expected outcomes. Remember, toxicity is not limited to the colon but is found throughout the body especially in fatty tissue, joints, arteries, the liver, muscles, and where there is inflammation.

By cleansing the colon, the elimination of toxins from the lungs, skin, kidneys, and liver will be enhanced and common signs of toxicity such as headaches, backaches, fatigue, lethargy, halitosis, skin conditions, irritability, and all the associated conditions found in the colon will be improved.

Every system in the body is connected to the colon by reflex points. (See Figure 3, Reflex Points of the Colon). **The action of the water and gentle massage will affect the corresponding parts of the body therapeutically.**

Treatments will usually last for **45 minutes.** Allow one-and-a-half hours for the initial consultation and an hour for subsequent treatments. (Incidentally, but also importantly, there is some evidence to show the use of laxatives can create a dependency. There is no evidence to show that colon hydrotherapy is habit forming.) Note, that as an organ the colon is in continuous use and is therefore rarely, if ever, completely empty. **The role of colonic hydrotherapy is not simply to empty the bowel, but with water entering and flushing its length is to produce a well-functioning bowel.**

During a treatment it is possible to cleanse the full length of the large intestine (unlike an enema which only reaches the lower part of the colon). A loss of friendly bacteria will be compensated for by taking **probiotics,** supplements that contain 'friendly' bacteria which are normally present in the digestive tract (*Bifidobacterium, Lactobacillus acidophilusi* and *Streptococcus faecium*, not to be confused with *S. faecalis* which is a possible pathogenic bacteria).

Probiotics are defined as non-pathogenic microbes that when ingested exert a positive influence on the health or physiology of the host. Studies in children have shown that probiotic supplementation may reduce the severity of viral gastroenteritis and the likelihood of developing atopic disease (conditions provoked by allergens). Probiotics have been studied as therapy in irritable bowel syndrome (IBS) cases and small placebo-controlled studies suggest efficacy, although whether probiotics are effective in treating IBS remains a topic of controversy. (Bousavaros A, 2008)

Moreover, some Practitioners recommend separate **prebiotic** supplements that contain the nutrients that these bacteria require in order to thrive. The key prebiotic nutrients, often seen in prebiotic supplements, are fructo-obligosaccharides (short-chain fatty acids) and inulin (a fibre). Chicory root and Jerusalem artichoke are common sources. (E M Haas, 2006). Some supplement suppliers now **combine** prebiotic and probiotic formulae.

The cleansed bowel means that unfriendly bacteria have been removed and the acid and alkaline balance restored allowing healthy bacteria to thrive. Every part of the body will benefit. Good bacteria can only breed in a clean environment, that is, one absent of putrefaction and accompanying harmful bacteria.

Colon hydrotherapy can still take place during a menstrual period and may help relieve the cramping associated with menstruation.

Following a colon hydrotherapy treatment it is recommended that the Patient resumes their usual meal times, makes intelligent choices about food, and only consumes a moderate amount of whatever seems gentle and nourishing. Clearly, salads, soups, fruit, vegetables, and fruit and vegetable juices are advised. (See Table 9, After Treatment Self-Care).

Hygiene, Cross-infection Concerns, and Preventative Measures

One of the most critical aspects of clinical practice is concerned with matters associated with hygiene, contamination, cross-infection, and the serious sicknesses that can result if, as Practitioners, we are at all negligent in this area of our work.

Hygiene is now regarded as one of the most important performance criterion in healthcare practice. We know that hospital-acquired infections (HAIs) are regularly in the news, for example, methicillin-resistant *Staphylococcus aureus* (MRSA), *Escherichia coli* (a large and diverse group of bacteria), and *Clostridium difficile*. We hear about 'superbugs' that are resistant to antibiotic treatments; the need for infection control strategies; the necessity to ensure all surfaces, ledges, corners, and recesses are clean (dust can be contaminated with, for example, the MRSA organism); and the requirement for Practitioners to be very careful about proper hand washing in order to prevent any cross- infections arising.

Our colon hydrotherapy clinic is not a hospital. We are not dealing with a number of Patients in the same area. We are not dealing with lots of visitors, we are not trying to manage the various types of problems associated with infections following surgery, but **we are responsible for ensuring our clinic, equipment, and professional practice meets all regulatory and responsible health and hygiene requirements.**

Therefore, in emphasizing the need for us to be robust about such requirements let us briefly consider MRSA, *E. coli* and *C. difficile* bacteria.

MRSA is found on the skin of many individuals and seems to cause no major problems, and such persons are considered to be carriers of the organism. However, if the organism gets inside the body, for example, under the skin or into the lungs, it can cause infections such as boils or pneumonia. MRSA is used to describe those examples of this organism that are resistant to commonly used antibiotics. (Methicillin was an antibiotic used to treat staphylococcus infections). If the organism is on the skin it can be passed around by physical contact. Usually there is nothing to worry about unless the organism is passed to someone who is already ill at which point a more serious infection may occur.

E. coli is a bacteria that causes severe cramps and diarrhoea. It is the main cause of bloody diarrhoea; the symptoms are worse in children and older people, and especially in people who have another illness. The most common way of getting this infection is by eating contaminated food. The germ can be passed from person to person. If a person has this infection and fails to wash their hands well after going to the toilet they can give the germ to other people when surfaces are touched, hands are shaken.

C. difficile is also a cause of diarrhoea. This bacteria produces two toxins that are responsible for the diarrhoea and which damage the cells lining the bowel. In addition, the bacterium can cause spores that enable it to survive in the environment outside the body, for example on floors and around toilets. (Other causes of diarrhoea such as salmonella do not form spores). Abdominal pain and fever may also occur, and occasionally Patients may develop a severe form of the disease called 'pseudomembranous colitis', which is characterized by significant damage to the large intestines. This may lead to a grossly dilated bowel, possibly resulting in rupture or perforation.

Unlike some other causes of diarrhoea it is rare for *C. difficile* to spread to other parts of the body such as the bloodstream. This infection is usually acquired in hospital. Occasionally, usually in young children or in Patients who have recently been treated for the infection, large amounts of the toxin may be detected in faeces without producing symptoms in the Patient. The reason for this is unknown.

Note: The issue of hepatitis infection is frequently asked about.

Hepatitis is usually contracted through unsafe sexual activity and by drug addicts sharing needles. However, vaccination is recommended for healthcare workers. Hepatitis A, which is found in the faeces of someone infected is the most common of seven types of viral hepatitis. It only takes a tiny amount of faeces getting inside another person's mouth to cause hepatitis A infection. Hepatitis B is more likely to cause long-term illness and permanent liver damage if not treated, and is most commonly passed through the exchange of bodily fluids with an infected person. Hepatitis C, like other forms of hepatitis, causes inflammation of the liver, but is transferred primarily through the blood. If you are ever worried about splashes, spillages, or similar issues, then speaking to your own Doctor is suggested.

The foregoing examples remind us why it is essential to use disposable gloves and disposable specula/piping and why all hard surfaces must be cleaned and disinfected before and after each Patient. In particular, surfaces subject to soiling, for example, the toilet, toilet seat, flush handle, and door knobs.

We need to **be rigorous about cleaning every part of the clinic,** and the thorough washing of the hands before and after Patient contact is the most efficient infection control measure we can take. Hands are the principal route by which cross-infection occurs. **Handwashing is one of the most important procedures for preventing the spread of disease.** Therefore, hand-hygiene guidance is as follows:

Always wet hands before applying soap or antiseptic solutions, rinse and dry thoroughly, and apply a good hand cream regularly. Open cuts or sores must be covered with a waterproof plaster and disposable gloves used. Nails must be kept short and clean and false nails or varnish must not be worn. The wearing of rings with ridges or stones is to be avoided as well as the wearing of watches or bracelets. Roll up long sleeves.

Liquid soap containing an emollient (an agent that soothes and softens the skin) must be available in all clinical and non-clinical areas for routine handwashing. Bar soap should not be used in clinical areas. Alcohol gel is useful on visibly clean hands. It is not a cleansing agent but can be used when rapid hand disinfection is required. It must be available in the clinic itself and used after a routine hand wash as an adequate method of decontaminating the hands and is sufficient for the procedure of colon hydrotherapy.

Wash hands using soap and running water for 10-15 seconds. The same applies for washing with aqueous antiseptic solutions, alcohol handrubs, gels, or wipes. (When applying alcohol gel, allow it to dry naturally on the skin).

Note: The use of gloves in addition to the process of hand-washing gives added protection, whereas the use of gloves as an alternative to handwashing may lead to infection. Needless to say, single use latex examination gloves must be used for all treatments. Latex finger cots or preferably a latex glove must be used for rectal examinations and then discarded.

A suitable lubricant must be used for speculum insertion with the necessary care to prevent the risk of cross-contamination. (Check with your Patient for any allergy to latex and if necessary use non-latex-based disposable examination gloves).

Hands should always be washed after removing **gloves** and before sterile gloves are worn. Gloves are for single use and must be changed between Patients and disposed of appropriately. Hands are to be dried using an air dryer or disposable paper towel. All **gowns, wraps, and paper,** or other coverings (for example, treatment-couch coverings) must be clean and in good repair. Practitioners must always be tidy and wear clean protective clothing, which must never be used to wipe hands.

Note: Disinfectants do not sterilize, they only reduce the number of some microbes. Nevertheless, they are essential for cleansing the colonic machine, and wiping down the treatment couch and surfaces in the clinic. It is recommended to use bleach for dealing with spillages of body fluids; detergent and water for general cleaning and wiping down. Faecal matter, blood, and vomit clearly pose a health risk and must be cleaned up immediately. The following procedure is recommended:

Put on disposable gloves and cover the spillage with paper towels. Pour bleach on the spillage and then wipe up with towels and dispose of accordingly. Discard gloves and wash hands thoroughly.

It is always best to adopt optimum hygiene practice at all times for the safety of Patients, self, and others who may frequent your clinic. Practitioners should always be clean and look clean, tidy, and smart. All the above guidelines are intended to assist in the avoidance of potential infections, and reflect a proper care of Patients.

Note: A 'Dirty Hands' study was conducted in 2008, for the first Global Hand-washing Day, at five train stations across England. Commuters were swab-tested for bacteria and the results analysed by the London School of Hygiene and Tropical Medicine. Contrary to the myth, that men are casual about hygiene, women were found to be three times more likely to have dirty hands than men. The bacteria found were all from the gut indicating that hands had not been washed properly. If a person is suffering from a diarrhoeal disease the potential for it to be passed on is increased significantly by failure to wash hands properly after going to the toilet. The message is simple; make sure you always wash your hands after using the toilet!!

Colon Hydrotherapy Machines and Treatment Facilities

Colon hydrotherapy requires **reliable and effective machines** that have been **designed for the purpose.** The use of machines that provide the highest possible guarantee of safety and hygiene is mandatory (See Useful Addresses). It seems that the core specifications are relatively common among the manufacturers. Nevertheless, with this in mind, it is essentially up to Practitioners to satisfy themselves as to the efficiency of given machines; consider such factors as cost and after-sales service; ease of installation and adherence to Local Authority specifications; ease of operation; display panel features and their value to you as the Practitioner; and the suitability and availability of the disposable items, and so on.

Colon Hydrotherapy machines include: the Colon Hydromat, which is manufactured by Hermann Apparatebau GmbH in Germany, Tanscom, and Dotolo, manufactured in Spain and the USA, respectively, and Gravity-Feed machines are also available.

Each of the producers manufacture models with different specifications. In addition, as noted, it is also possible to purchase systems where the water is gravity-feed, again see Useful Addresses. Clearly, the chosen equipment must be fitted and plumbed-in, according to the manufacturer's instructions and must meet Local Authority public health requirements. Water temperatures must be strictly adhered to and ALL systems must be fitted with a suitable water filter which MUST be replaced following use, according to the **manufacturer's instructions.**

If gravity-feed equipment is being used, the feed tank, enema bucket, associated piping, and Y-connector should be frequently disinfected, at least weekly. (For detailed health and safety guidance on the use of gravity-feed systems Practitioners are advised to liaise with the Association and Register of Colon Hydrotherapists (ARCH) and refer to their Treatment Facilities, A Guide to Good Practice). Again, installation instructions must be followed to the letter.

The layout of **the treatment room** will of course be determined by its size and shape. The aim is to ensure enough space for comfort and purpose where there is room enough for the colon hydrotherapy machine and equipment; room for the treatment couch (a fully adjustable couch is recommended in order to facilitate easy access for different size Patients); hand basin (for the Therapist's use); desk; and chairs. Immediately off the room will be the toilet (for use of Patients during working hours only); hand basin and medicated soap (with paper towels, hand-wipes, hand dryer); waste bin (for the disposal of sanitary towels and soiled articles); and space for changing. Clean towels or gowns, for each Patient, will be provided as well as pegs for hanging clothes.

The toilet and treatment room must be properly ventilated and all surfaces must be easily cleanable. Without exception, the treatment-room floor surface/covering must be washable and impervious to water, and walls/ceilings also to be of surfaces that are easy to clean. Disposable specula, any piping, and any other soiled materials must be disposed of in accordance with Local Authority regulations, which may require the use and collection from the 'yellow bag' biohazard service. THE USE OF DISPOSABLE EQUIPMENT ONLY is, without question, advocated.

The treatment room should be warm and heated (or cooled in the summertime) using properly installed equipment certified by an approved electrician.

A waiting room with a separate toilet is essential allowing Patients to wait in comfort and also, if they so choose, to rest after treatment, and to be offered a drink before leaving.

The Gastrointestinal Tract and Motility

On average the bowel is 1.5m (5 feet) in length and 6.5cm (2.5 inches) in diameter. It extends from the ileum to the anus.

Few of us give much thought to our bowel except on the occasions we need to empty, or at other times when we feel discomfort. Yet one in four adults in the UK will suffer from bowel problems or disorders. A poor diet is the main cause of problems, that is, diets which are high in meat, sugar, fat, and are low in fibre. Hence, **poor bowel management is at the root of the majority of health problems.**

Examples in support of this statement include: clogging of the arteries (atherosclerosis), clogging of the joints (arthritis and rheumatism), and clogging of the colon (constipation, spastic colon, diverticulosis, IBS). Although colon hydrotherapy is not a cure on its own of such diseases, it will ensure a cleansed bowel for us. By cleansing the colon, the whole body system is significantly aided (See Figure 5, The Main Diseases of the Digestive Tract).

Toxaemia results from the absorption of certain chemicals. Conjugation (a normal liver function where many toxic substances are made less harmful) is obstructed when the body's major systems of elimination are overtaxed, or have a significant degree of dysfunction, and as such adds to intestinal putrefaction.

Moreover, we also know that nervous **tension and stress** causes contraction in all the orifices of the body which makes motility and the efficient elimination of toxic materials difficult. Much of our stress will be experienced through a nervous and upset stomach, which is often a reflection of difficulties that lie further down in the alimentary canal. **Intestinal toxaemia** results in systemic autointoxication.

Symptoms associated with autointoxication include: headaches of various types, back pain, depression, drowsiness, bloating, fatigue, skin conditions, abdominal pain, sinus problems, erratic heartbeats, bad breath, catarrh, insomnia, arthritis, hyper/hypo blood pressure, itching, and leg pains.

Intestinal toxaemia manifests itself, for example, as follows: fatigue; lower-back pain; nervousness; sciatica; gastrointestinal conditions; the malabsorption of nutrients; allergies; skin condition; asthma; endocrine disturbances; diseases of eye, ear, and throat; neurocirculatory abnormalities; cardiac irregularities; headaches; arthritis; pathological changes in the breasts. All these conditions have responded to therapy for intestinal toxaemia. (Jensen B, 1999).

Thus it is established that a relationship exists between intestinal toxaemia and abnormal cellular function. **Pathology, it is suggested, could be defined as abnormal function. Therefore, good health is as much a function of our elimination status as the quality of the food we ingest.**

Pathology results when toxins are present in such numbers that they cannot be dealt with by the liver. Colon hydrotherapy effectively removes stagnant faecal material from the colon wall, preventing any build up of these toxins, resulting in a reduced load on the liver and other vital organs.

Food should pass through the body approximately every eighteen hours. Any delay due to the effects of fermentation, clogging or limited movements will effect the rest of the body. **Take care of the bowel and every organ will respond** accordingly. Remember that as toxins accumulate in the tissues changes in cellular functions take place, particularly in the tissues in which the toxins have settled. The body becomes fatigued, and tired bodies reduce their capacity to throw off toxins. Therefore, detoxification starts with the bowel and so often disease also!

As quoted by Jensen (1999), Dr W A Lane, 1856–1943, (who later became the Royal Surgeon), defined chronic intestinal stasis (the stagnation or cessation of flow, when for example intestinal contents are obstructed thus hindering onward movement, i.e. peristalsis) as an "abnormal delay in transmission of intestinal contents; delay allows multiplication of undesirable organisms and the subsequent development of toxaemia; this leads to progressive degenerative changes in every tissue and a definite and unmistakable series of symptoms."

Food transit times (See Figure 2, Food Transit Times), are the length of time food stays in each segment of the digestive system. **The term 'motility' is used to describe the ability of the digestive tract to propel its contents** and is summarized as follows: in the mouth a few seconds/minutes, (remember the value of chewing food thoroughly before swallowing) in the oesophagus four to eight seconds, in the stomach two to five hours, in the small intestine three to five hours, in the large intestine 10 hours (to several days).

Ideally by 10pm breakfast residue has been discharged via a bowel movement at bedtime. The lunch residue is moving through the colon and the dinner residue is waiting to enter the colon. The lower end of the large intestine is of a size that requires emptying every six hours but by habit we retain its contents 24 hours. The result is ulcer and cancer.

The gastrointestinal tract is divided into four distinct parts, and each is discussed at length below: the oesophagus, stomach, small intestine, and large intestine (the colon). They are separated from each other by special muscles called sphincters that stay tightly closed and regulate, as necessary, food contents from one part to another. Each part has a unique function to perform in digestion and as a consequence has a distinct motility. When usual motility is disturbed, symptoms such as bloating, vomiting, diarrhoea, and constipation result.

1. The **normal motility and function of the oesophagus** (or gullet), which extends from the pharynx to the cardiac sphincter (controlled by the vagus nerve), is simply to transport food from the mouth to the stomach. When a mouthful of food has been masticated and well mixed with saliva, the movement of the tongue and cheeks convert it into a soft rounded mass called a **bolus**. The bolus is grasped in the pharynx by the contraction of the constrictor muscles and forced into the oesophagus. (At the same time the larynx is raised and the epiglottis acts as a guard to its upper opening, the trachea).

There are three pairs of **salivary glands,** (the parotid, submandibular, and sublingual glands), with saliva being the mixed secretion of each, which **is alkaline** in reaction and contains the enzyme ptyalin that converts into a sugar called maltose. Saliva also moistens the food and acts as a lubricant aiding the act of swallowing and passage of food down the oesophagus.

So, the act of **swallowing**, though more or less automatic, is a deliberate and voluntary one. Thereafter, the individual has no further control and it becomes involuntary, a reflex action. This is a protective reflex preventing the aspiration of food into the respiratory tract. The whole process of swallowing takes about 10 to 20 seconds and the muscular contraction is called peristalsis.

Peristalsis may be defined as a wave of muscular contraction preceded by a wave of relaxation that causes the content of a hollow tube to be passed onwards. The cardiac sphincter muscle opens so that the food we swallow can enter the stomach and then normally stays tightly closed in order to prevent acid in the stomach from washing up into the oesophagus thus avoiding reflux from occurring when the stomach contracts. When acid washes up into the oesophagus, due to a weak sphincter muscle or hiatus hernia, irritation of the lining of the oesophagus occurs: heartburn. A hiatus hernia weakens the sphincter.

Ineffective swallowing is called **dysphagia,** sometimes the result of disease or stroke, which can cause food to back up in the oesophagus causing vomiting. Sometimes Patients have pain or discomfort (unlike heartburn) which may be confused with pain from the heart and comes from spastic contractions or muscle spasm. The test that is used to find the cause is oesophageal **manometry,** which is the measurement of pressure within organs or to indicate muscular activity in motile tubes such as the oesophagus, rectum, or bile duct.

2. The **stomach** is a J-shaped structure which lies in the upper part of the abdominal cavity and forms a receptacle for the bolus after its passage down the oesophagus. The bolus mixes with digestive juices so that nutrients can be absorbed when reaching the small intestine. Therefore, the **primary functions** of the stomach are: to store food ingested during the meal and then to regulate its release into the duodenum; to churn and mix food with secretions and gastric juice of the stomach; and secretion of the intrinsic factor, (for B12 absorption). Carbohydrate foods pass from the stomach soon after digestion and require half the time required by proteins to pass.

Motility of the stomach involves three types of contractions known as mixing waves, as follows:

- Rhythmic waves, three per minute, synchronized contractions, in the lower part of the stomach (pyloric antrum), which create waves of food particles and gastric juice to 'splash' against the closed sphincter muscle, the pyloric sphincter, to 'grind' the food down into smaller particles. The pylorus then relaxes at intervals and allows small quantities of food to enter the duodenum. This food is now in a semi-liquid state and this partially digested material is called **chyme**

- The upper part of the stomach shows slow relaxations, lasting a minute or more, these follow each swallow, which then allows food to enter the stomach. At other times the upper part of the stomach shows slow contractions which help to empty the stomach. The time taken to empty the stomach will of course depend on the nature, digestibility, and quantity of food taken.

- The consumption of an ordinary meal takes about five hours to leave the stomach. Between meals, after all the digestible food has left the stomach, there are occasional bursts of very strong, synchronized contractions that are accompanied by opening the pyloric sphincter muscle thus moving any indigestible particles out of the stomach and into the duodenum, the first part of the small intestine.

Peristaltic movements taking place in an empty stomach give rise to the sensation of hunger. Moreover, the diaphragm pushes the stomach downward with each inspiration, and pulls it upward, each expiration.

Delayed gastric emptying, (gastroparesis) including nausea and vomiting may happen for several reasons: the stomach outlet at the pylorus and duodenum may be obstructed by an ulcer, tumour, or something large and indigestible; the pyloric sphincter may not open enough at the required times to allow food to pass through, due to a nerve-dependent reflex that may sometimes become damaged; the normally rhythmic, three per minute contractions of the lower part of the stomach become disorganized so that the contents of the stomach are not pushed towards the pyloric sphincter. This usually has a neurological basis, the most common cause being type 2 diabetes. (The term diabetes mellitus is being replaced by the use of the term type 2 diabetes). Nevertheless, in many cases the cause of delayed gastric emptying is unknown (idiopathic). (The pyloric valve ensures liquids usually pass through in advance of the bolus. The valve secretes alkaline liquid containing pepsin. It is the combination of pepsin and hydrochloric acid inside of the stomach that helps liquefy solid proteins).

Also, some Patients will speak of pain or discomfort being felt in the centre of their abdomen, just above their naval. It is estimated that around a third of these Patients have delayed gastric emptying and a further third show a failure of relaxation in the upper stomach after swallowing, known as 'abnormal gastric accommodation reflex'. About half of Patients with such symptoms also have a sensitive or irritable stomach, which causes sensations of discomfort when the stomach is filled with even small amounts. (Wellsprings College of Colon Hydrotherapy, 2007).

In many cases the Patient will do better with **digestive enzyme supplements**, which is a subject discussed later in this section.

The inner lining of the stomach is the **mucous membrane** which contains the glands that secrete the gastric juice. The mucous membrane is 'thrown' into folds (rugae) thereby increasing the total surface area of the stomach from which secretion can take place. This secretion is continuous, even when the stomach is at rest, for example, during the hours before breakfast, there is always some gastric juice present.

The stomach wall is impermeable to the passage of most materials in blood hence most substances are not absorbed until they reach the small intestine. The stomach does absorb some water, electrolytes (atoms that conduct electricity), certain drugs (especially aspirin), and alcohol.

Gastric juice is a clear watery fluid and, in contrast to saliva, **is acid** in reaction. The average adult produces approximately 2l of gastric juice per day. The acidity is due to the presence of hydrochloric acid (HCL) secreted by the glands of the gastric mucosa. The intake of food into the stomach is followed by a considerable increase in the output of gastric juice, partly as a reflex mechanism through the **vagus nerve** and partly by means of a chemical messenger, the hormone called **gastrin.** The psychological stimuli of sight and smell also cause a flow of gastric juice similar to the effect on the salivary glands.

The chemical composition of gastric juice is as follows:

- **Mucous,** which coats and protects the epithelial cells that line the stomach, consists mainly of mucin, a glycoprotein (proteins combined with a carbohydrate). Mucous also acts as a lubricant and a carrier of enzymes.

- **Pepsinogen**, which, when activated by HCL, begins the first stage of the chemical digestion of protein by making the stomach enzyme pepsin. Pepsin then converts protein into less complex substances called peptones. (Further stages of protein digestion take place in the small intestine).

- **HCL,** secreted by the parietal cells of the gastric glands in the fundic region of the stomach, sterilizes chyme and activates pepsinogen.

79

- **The secretion** of the **intrinsic factor,** a glycoprotein, which is necessary for the absorption of vitamin B12. Failure of secretion leads to a deficiency in the body of the vitamin, and development of the condition pernicious anaemia.

Remember that vitamins also help to convert macronutrients, (carbohydrates, protein, and fats), into metabolically useful forms, by acting as co-enzymes in collaboration with enzymes. (See Table 6, Enzymes: A Summary).

Before we move to discussing transit times of the small intestine, let us consider the matter of **digestive enzyme supplements,** which are often recommended by Practitioners as part of a treatment plan, and because they enter the small intestine by the pancreatic duct at the duodenum and mix with the foods that have left the stomach. (See also 'Diet and Nutrition' section)

We know that enzymes are complex protein molecules, and that the body contains around 1,300 different enzymes, which breakdown nutrients, rebuild cells, and have a great effect upon the immune system. We also know that the pancreatic enzymes amylase, lipase, and trypsin assist in the breakdown of starches, fats, and proteins.

Digestive enzyme supplements include pancreatic enzymes, plant-derived enzymes, and fungal-derived enzymes. There are three classes: proteolytic enzymes needed to digest protein; lipase needed to digest fat; and amylases needed to digest carbohydrates. Supplementing the diet with digestive enzymes can make a real difference to a Patient's digestive health. For example: indigestion, heartburn, irregularity, gas, bloating, and constipation are often the result of inadequate enzymes.

Moreover, supplements are likely to include bromelain (an enzyme found in pineapple), and papain (an enzyme found in the papaya fruit) which, respectively, act as anti-inflammatory agents and aid nutrient absorption. The goal is to achieve, as soon as possible, normal digestion, assimilation, and elimination in order to ensure appropriate motility. (DeFelice, 2006).

3. The small intestine is the portion of the alimentary tract extending from the pyloric sphincter of the stomach to its termination in the first part of the large intestine called the caecum at the ileoceacal sphincter (valve). It consists of three parts: the **duodenum, jejunum, and ileum.**

The duodenum is fixed to the posterior abdominal wall by the peritoneum and is the shortest part of the small intestine, about 25cm (10 inches). About halfway along the duodenum the bile duct and the pancreatic duct enter together at a small papilla (a nipple shaped protuberance) called the 'ampulla of Vater'. The jejunum is 2.5m (8 feet) long and the final portion of the small intestine, the ileum, measures about 3.6m (12 feet) are partially moveable within the abdominal cavity. Although given separate names, the former passes into the latter about two-fifths of the way down the course of the small intestine.

Since almost all the digestion and **absorption of nutrients** occurs in the small intestine its structure is especially adapted for this function. Each villus contains capillaries into which are absorbed the products of carbohydrate and protein digestion (glucose and amino acids) and a central lymphatic vessel or lacteal into which fats are absorbed. Villi are finger-like processes that project from some membranous surfaces. Numerous intestinal villi line the small intestine. As noted, each contains a network of blood capillaries and lacteal. Their function is to absorb the products of digestion and they greatly increase the surface area over which this can take place.

As in the stomach the mucous membrane is arranged in folds thus greatly increasing the surface from which secretion and absorption can take place. The mucous membrane contains glands that secrete intestinal juices; and lymphatic tissue is found in the submucous layer in solitary nodes or in collected masses (often several centimetres long) called Peyer's Patches that are present in the lower part of the ileum.

Motility of the small intestine, during and after a meal, shows very **irregular contractions that move the food content back and forth and mixes it with the digestive enzymes.** The contractions are unsynchronized but move the contents slowly towards the large intestine.

It normally takes around 90 to 120 minutes for the first part of a meal to reach the large intestine and the last portion of the meal may take five hours to reach the large intestine. This pattern of motility is called the 'fed (or eating) pattern'. Two other kinds of motility seen in the small intestine are: brief but clustered contractions, lasting for only several seconds, occurring mostly in the upper part of the small intestine. These are synchronized peristaltic movements, and secondly, is the giant migrating contraction that occurs in the lower part of the small intestine, the ileum, and it is peristaltic over longer distances.

Abnormal motility patterns in the small intestine can result from intestinal blockage causing pain, bloating, nausea, and vomiting. Abnormalities in the intestinal muscle may cause the intestine to balloon out so that contractions of the muscle are unable to move contents forward. Note: bacterial overgrowth in the small intestine can be the result of poor motility in that part of the alimentary canal with bacteria consuming the nutrients before these are absorbed!

4. Motility of the colon. Following a meal there is a **gastro-ilea reflex** in which ilea peristalsis is intensified and any chyme in the ileum is forced into the caecum. Movements of the colon start when substances enter through the ileocaecal sphincter and accumulate in the ascending colon. Initially, contractions mix the contents of the large intestine back and forth; however, these contractions do not move the chyme forward. This process of **back and forth movement** provides for the re-absorption of water, thus preventing the body from becoming dehydrated. (Between what we drink and what is secreted by the stomach and small intestine in order to facilitate the absorption of nutrients around 22l of fluid enter the large intestine daily).

A further characteristic movement of the large intestine is **haustral churning,** which involves the filling, distension, and contraction of haustra and the movement of chyme from one haustrum to the next. Peristalsis also occurs, although at a slower pace, than in other portions of the gastrointestinal tract.

An **essential motility** is the **'high-amplitude propagating contraction'.** In healthy people, these contractions only occur six to eight times per day. These contractions are extremely strong and begin in the first part of the large intestine and sweep all the way to the rectum, stopping just above the rectum. A final movement is **mass peristalsis,** which is a strong peristaltic wave beginning at about the middle of the transverse colon and driving the contents of the colon into the rectum.

The resulting distension of the rectal wall stimulates pressure-sensitive receptors that cause impulses to be sent along the nerves to the spinal chord and subsequently to the brain, where the conscious sensation to defecate is aroused, in other words, initiating a reflex to defecate. If this call is neglected the rectum accommodates itself to its contents by relaxation of the muscles in its walls, impulses cease to travel along the nerves, and the desire to eliminate passes off.

As we are now aware it is the arrival of more faecal matter into the rectum that will cause further distension and another set of impulses concerning motility are conveyed to the nervous system and again producing the conscious desire to evacuate the bowel. Failure to respond to this natural process is a common form of constipation and the harder the contents of the rectum will become.

The act of defecation is a reflex in the infant. In the adult is under the control of the will. The following actions occur:

- The sphincter muscle of the anus relaxes.
- The muscle walls of the rectum contract.
- The muscles of the floor of the pelvis contract.
- The pressure within the abdomen is raised: by holding the breath and contracting the diaphragm and by contracting the muscles of the abdominal wall. (Alternatively, my yoga tutor taught that it is potentially a less forceful action to exhale in

order to defecate as the stomach muscles are pulled in and therefore automatically raise the diaphragm.)

Remember, that a number of these motility actions are increased in force if the squatting posture is adopted, this being the natural and primitive posture. Also by holding one's hands in the air above the head, thus increasing pressure in the abdominal cavity, further assists the ability to defecate. It is the injection of water into the rectum by the colon hydrotherapist that has the effect of rapidly distending its walls that initiates the mechanism whereby the desire to defecate is produced. The water also helps soften and break up hard masses of faeces. Stools will be discussed in the section 'The Five Systems of Elimination'.

Diseases of the Colon

The main diseases of the colon are: polyps and benign growths, diverticulitis, ulcerative colitis, Crohn's disease, and colorectal cancer, which is cancer of the colon and rectum. (See Figure 5, Main Diseases of the Digestive Tract).

A polyp is a benign (non-cancerous) growth on the lining of the colon, and can be from 2mm to 5cm or more in diameter. Commonly, the abnormal cells form a small ball (about the size of a pea) on the end of a stalk of normal cells.

The type of cell that forms the polyp varies and is important in determining the polyp's potential for developing into a cancer. Metaplastic polyps have almost no risk of becoming malignant. However, adenomatous polyps, which are similar in appearance to metaplastic polyps, are the next most common polyps and do have the potential to become malignant.

Most polyps result from some form of genetic (DNA) mutation. (Even in a healthy adult's colon about 10% of the lining cells contain major abnormalities).

Fortunately, almost all these cells seem to undergo a form of programmed death called apoplosis and then fall off harmlessly into bowel cavity, the lumen.

Polyps usually cause no symptoms until they grow to 2cm or more in diameter. Then the most common symptom is bleeding from the anus. Blood might be noticed on underwear, on the toilet paper following bowel movement, or in the stool. Blood can make the stool look black, or it can show up as red streaks in the stool.

Constipation or diarrhoea lasting more than a week can occur, and if the Patient has any of these symptoms a doctor should be consulted in order to establish the nature of the problem. Polyps can lead to severe colicky pain and can cause profuse watery diarrhoea, which can then result in severe potassium deficiency causing muscle weakness.

Polyps can be seen during colonoscopy (a telescopic examination of the whole of the bowel starting at the rectum). Most polyps can be removed whilst the Patient is sedated, during a colonoscopy. With sigmoidoscopy the doctor puts a thin flexible tube into the rectum to examine the final third of the colon. Other investigative methods include a barium enema (a liquid called barium is placed into the rectum) before an X-ray is taken. Barium makes the intestines appear white in the X-ray picture, polyps are dark so can be easily seen, and a digital examination can also be used to check the rectum.

Dietary changes have so far proved ineffective at preventing polyps. However, it is believed a person is more likely to develop polyps if they smoke, eat fatty foods, drink alcohol, weigh too much, and fail to exercise. Therefore, lower the risk of polyps by doing the opposite and eat more fruit and vegetables!

A benign growth (also known as benign mass, benign neoplasm, or benign tumour) is basically a non-recurring tumour (when surgically removed) and does not spread to other parts of the body. A tumour is a mass of tissue that serves no useful purpose and generally exists at the expense of healthy tissue. Benign tumours tend to grow more slowly than malignant tumours and are less likely to cause health problems.

However, that does not mean we can just forget about them. Remember, colon polyps are benign tumours and but most colon cancer develops from polyps. That is why colon cancer screening is so important. As we have noted a colonoscopy can identify and remove benign tumours growing in the colon.

Diverticulitis is a condition in which the **diverticuli in the colon rupture.** This results in infection in the tissues that surround the colon. Pressure within the colon causes bulging pockets of tissue (sacs) that push out from the colon walls. A small bulging sac pushing out from the colon wall is called a diverticulum. More than one bulging sac is referred to as **diverticula.** Diverticula can occur throughout the colon but are most common near the end of the part of the colon called the sigmoid. **Note: the condition of having these diverticula in the colon is called diverticulosis. A Patient with diverticulosis may have few or no symptoms,** but some will develop bleeding, constipation, abdominal cramps, and colon obstruction. When a diverticulum becomes infected and ruptures (bursting apart) the condition is called diverticulitis.

A Patient suffering from diverticulitis will have abdominal pain, tenderness, and fever. When bleeding originates from a diverticulum it is called diverticular bleeding. A Patient who suffers from diverticulosis in the colon is referred to as having diverticular disease. Less common signs or symptoms are vomiting, bloating, frequent urination, difficulty or pain while urinating, bleeding from the rectum, and tenderness in the abdomen when wearing a belt or when bending over.

This disease is common in developed countries but rare in Asia and Africa. Diverticular disease increases with age. It is uncommon before the age of 40 and is seen in more than 15% of people (in the USA) over the age of 60.

Treatment of diverticulitis depends on the severity of the symptoms and how many acute episodes the Patient has experienced. If symptoms are mild, a liquid or low-fibre diet and antibiotics may be recommended.

Those at risk of complications, or are experiencing recurrent attacks of diverticulitis, may require surgery to remove the diseased portion of the colon and reconnect the healthy segments of the colon, called sigmoid resection. In cases when the colon is so inflamed and the Patient may be experiencing a life-threatening infection, resection with colostomy may be performed. In such procedures the colostomy is usually temporary until the infection and inflammation clear. (To create a colostomy the surgeon makes an opening in the abdominal wall. The colon is then brought out through the opening and waste passes through the opening into a bag).

Diverticular disease results, essentially, from eating a diet low in fibre.

Fibre is the part of fruits, vegetables, and grains that the body cannot digest, therefore it passes through the intestines pretty much unchanged, softening the stools and aiding their elimination. (Soluble and insoluble fibre helps prevent constipation).

Without fibre, stools are dry and small, and the intestinal muscles must contract with greater force to pass the stools along the colon, thus generating a higher pressure in the colon. The excess pressure leads to weak spots in the colon wall that eventually bulge out to form sacs/pouches, the diverticula. The sigmoid area of the colon is subject to the highest amount of pressure because it is the narrowest portion of the colon. Constipation is the main cause of the increased pressure.

Ulcerative colitis means inflammation of the colon's lining (the mucosa) and always involves the rectum as well as parts of the colon. When the disease affects only the rectum it is known as **proctitis**. An ulcer is a break in the skin that fails to heal and is accompanied by inflammation, which may bleed and can cause frequent bouts of watery diarrhoea that may contain blood and mucous. Ulcerative colitis can also cause lower abdominal cramping pain, bloating, and increased abdominal gas. (The other main inflammatory bowel disease, Crohn's disease, can affect any part of the alimentary canal, from the mouth to the anus).

About one in 1000 people develop ulcerative colitis. Its cause is unknown although possible suggestions include: an abnormal response by the body's immune system to normal intestinal bacteria thus causing inflammation, and heredity, that is, passed to child from parent if they are suffering from the disease.

About one in five people with ulcerative colitis have a close relative who also has it, so there may be a genetic factor. Other causes may be certain foods and drugs, antibiotics disrupting the normal balance of bacteria in the bowel. For example, *C. difficile* **colitis** occurs when the spores of the bacteria remain dormant in the colon until the person takes an antibiotic. The antibiotic disrupts the other bacteria living in the colon that prevent *C. difficile* from transforming into its active disease-causing bacterial form, which then produces toxic chemicals that inflame and damage the colon. The chemicals kill the tissue of the inner lining of the colon, the tissue falls off, is mixed with white blood cells (pus) and gives the appearance of a white membranous patch covering the lining of the colon. (*C. difficile* spores are found frequently in hospitals and nursing homes). (MedicineNet, October 2008)

When ulcerative colitis affects more of the colon, the symptoms become more severe and may include: pain on opening the bowels; urgent and frequent need to open the bowels; the sensation of incomplete emptying of the bowels; diarrhoea even during the night; nausea (the feeling that one is about to vomit); loss of appetite; weight loss; and extreme tiredness.

The aim of treatment is to control flare-ups as quickly as possible and to reduce the chance of further flare-ups. Steroids act quickly to dampen down inflammation (5-aminosalicylate medicine is used as an alternative to steroids). Approximately one-third of sufferers require surgery. The colon is removed and the small intestine is joined to the anus. A pouch is made from the small intestine to act as a replacement rectum.

Having this disease can be physically and emotionally very stressful. Frequent bouts of diarrhoea can easily interfere with work and normal social activities. Nevertheless for most people with ulcerative colitis remission from the disease can be maintained for very long periods of time allowing a normal family and working life.

Crohn's disease (an autoimmune disorder) is also an inflammatory bowel disease that, like diverticulitis and ulcerative colitis, can have both acute (short-term) and chronic (long-term) effects. As noted, Crohn's disease may affect any part of the digestive system, from the mouth to the anus. It is most common in the lower part of the small intestine or the first part of the large intestine. It often affects more than one part of the bowel leaving normal and unaffected areas in-between.

When the lower sections of the bowel are the main areas affected it is not easy to distinguish from ulcerative colitis. Crohn's disease affects about one in every 1,500 people, mostly adults, with slightly more women than men being affected. The exact cause is not known but it is thought that the body's immune system overreacts to a virus or bacterium causing ongoing inflammation.

People with Crohn's disease have an increased blood flow in the wall of the bowel so that it becomes swollen. This can also cause inflammation and ulceration.

Moreover, smoking increases the risk of Crohn's disease and it is more likely to be found in people who eat a high sugar and low-fibre diet. Once started the disease tends to be a life-long condition.

The symptoms include: diarrhoea (up to 20 times during a 24-hour period) which may contain blood and mucous; pain (often described as colicky or cramping) felt anywhere in the abdomen that may be sore to touch and swollen; loss of appetite; weight loss (diarrhoea can of course lead to weight loss); people with the disease may at times have a high temperature; rectal bleeding, which may be serious and persistent, and can lead to anaemia; painful fissures (tears) and ulceration or abscesses (pus-filled areas) around the anus.

Active Crohn's disease may also cause problems in the rest of the body, such as mouth ulcers, pain in the joints, eye inflammation, and rashes (tender red lumps called erythema nodosum) or ulcers (called pyoderma) on the skin.

Although there is no cure for Crohn's disease, symptoms can improve with dietary changes, drugs, or surgery, or a combination of these. An elemental diet (a liquid diet, made up of simple forms of protein, carbohydrates, and fats, which can be absorbed without further digestion) may be recommended when the disease is active and can cause a remission of the disease. If there is narrowing of the bowel, a low residue diet (one low in fibre) may be recommended. When food is not being absorbed well a low-fat diet may be recommended.

For people with major complications short periods of parenteral feeding (through a route other than the mouth, usually by injection into a vein) in hospital may be needed. For the rest of the time it is important for people with the disease to eat a balanced diet with high-fibre content. Vitamin and iron supplements are often necessary as these nutrients may not be properly absorbed from the bowel.

Colorectal cancer, also called colon cancer or bowel cancer, includes cancerous growths in the colon, rectum, and appendix. It is the third most common form of cancer and the second leading cause of cancer-related death in the developed world. Many colorectal cancers are thought to arise from adenomatous polyps in the colon.

Treatment is usually through surgery, which in many cases is followed by chemotherapy. Colorectal cancer often causes no symptoms until it has reached a relatively advanced stage. Periodic screening for the disease with faecal occult blood testing and colonoscopy is recommended. (Occult blood refers to blood not easily seen by the naked eye, blood that can only be detected microscopically or by chemical testing).

When symptoms occur they depend upon the site of the lesion. (A lesion is an area of tissue with impaired function due to injury or disease). Generally speaking the nearer the lesion is to the anus the more bowel symptoms there will be, such as: change in bowel habits (frequency, quality and consistency of stools, constipation, and/or diarrhoea); bloody stools or rectal bleeding; stools with mucous; melaena (black tarry faeces due to partly digested blood from higher up the digestive tract, for example, stomach, or duodenal disease); feeling of incomplete defecation (tenesmus, usually associated with rectal cancer); reduction in diameter of faeces; and bowel obstruction which is rare.

Constitutional symptoms include anaemia and a complete blood test will confirm a low haemoglobin level; anorexia (loss of appetite); asthenia (weakness or loss of strength); and unexplained weight loss.

The pathology of the tumour is usually determined from an analysis of tissue taken from a biopsy or surgery. Cancers on the right side (ascending colon and caecum grows outward from one location in the bowel wall. Left-side tumours tend to grow around the bowel, circumferentially like a napkin ring, and can cause obstruction. Colon cancer 'staging' is an estimate of the amount or extent of invasion including the degree of lymph-node involvement and whether there is distant metastasis (the spread of malignant tumour from its site of origin).

A diet high in red meat and low in fresh fruit, vegetables, and fish increases the risk of colorectal cancer. Chronic inflammation, as in inflammatory bowel disease, may predispose Patients to malignancy. Treatment depends on the staging of the cancer.

When colorectal cancer is diagnosed at early stages (with little spread) it can be curable. Surgery remains the primary treatment while chemotherapy and/or radiotherapy may be recommended depending on any other medical factors.

In summary, we arrive at a position where there is clarity regarding symptoms that cannot be overlooked by the Practitioner when considering the administration of a colon hydrotherapy treatment.

If, as a Practitioner, you have any doubts or concerns about progressing with a treatment in the light of specific concerns as to the appropriateness on medical grounds (and your own informed assessment), or, for other more general concerns, (for example, the emotional health of the Patient) then ask the Patient to seek from their Doctor a note and opinion confirming (or not confirming) the suitability of the Patient for the treatment being sought by them.

Symptoms not to be overlooked by the Practitioner and when Patients should be advised to speak to their Doctor are as follows:

- Chronic or persistent pain and/or tenderness.

- Chronic indigestion, diarrhoea, constipation.

- Alternating diarrhoea and constipation.

- Swelling or distension of the stomach.

- Wanting to move bowels and being unable to.

- Pale, ill-formed stools.

- Blood in stools.

- Unexplained weight loss.

Before we list the symptoms and conditions suitable, and generally considered safe for treatment, (**indications**), and those symptoms and conditions generally considered unsuitable (**contraindications**) it is important to clarify our understanding of other relevant diseases and syndromes.

Irritable Bowel Syndrome (IBS) is sometimes referred to by the misnomer of 'irritable bowel disease' causing confusion with the far more serious inflammatory conditions described in earlier paragraphs. IBS is not a disease but a syndrome. The term syndrome refers to a combination or mixture of signs, conditions, and symptoms which usually go together to form an often distinct picture or profile. Therefore, a syndrome is a mixture of symptoms. IBS is a mixture of abdominal symptoms for which there is no apparent cause. (See also 'Indications for Colon Hydrotherapy Treatment' below).

Coeliac disease (or gluten allergy) is a life-long condition of the small intestine. Gluten, found in wheat, barley, oats, and rye, is a mixture of two proteins, gliadin and glutenin. When combined with water gluten becomes sticky and forms dough. In coeliac disease, gluten causes the immune system to produce **antibodies** that attack and destroy the delicate lining, the villi, of the intestine which is responsible for absorbing nutrients from food, vitamins, folic acid, iron, and calcium. Coeliac disease is therefore an **autoimmune disorder**. (Antibodies are a special kind of blood protein that attack antigens, bacteria, pollen grains, foreign red blood cells, and are the basis of both immunity and allergy).

This results in nutrients going through the intestine without being absorbed (malabsorption), leading to diarrhoea, vitamin and mineral deficiencies, anaemia, and thin/brittle bones (osteoporosis). (There is also a condition known as coeliac sprue syndrome in which the villi atrophy, waste away, for unknown reasons).

Coeliac disease occurs in people who are genetically prone to it and can affect them at any age. Symptoms do not appear until **foods containing gluten are introduced into the diet.**

Symptoms in adults include: weight loss with pale, foul-smelling diarrhoea; constipation and abdominal bloating with wind. However, around half of adults do not have these symptoms but speak to their doctor about extreme tiredness (a sign of anaemia), psychological problems like depression; bone pain and sometimes fractures (due to the thinning of the bones); ulcers in the mouth; and a blistering, itchy skin rash mostly on the elbows and knees, called dermatitis herpetiformis.

Blood tests will detect antibodies found in coeliac disease. An endoscopy and biopsy of a specimen of the small intestine lining will confirm diagnosis from the examination of the size and shape of the villi. It is usual to repeat the test after several months on a gluten-free diet in order to check that the lining has recovered. Damage will be caused as soon as gluten is eaten again.

Therefore, it is not possible to prevent coeliac disease but gluten-free substitutes are readily available from most supermarkets, as well as recipe books! There is no gluten in fruit, salads, vegetables, potatoes, rice, maize, nuts, chicken meat, fish, eggs, and dairy products.

Whipple's Disease is a rare infectious disease that typically infects the bowel but occurs most often in the small intestine. An endoscopy of the duodenum and jejunum can show pale yellow mucosa with red patches that can cause lesions: tissue with impaired function. Therefore, not surprisingly, Whipples' disease causes malabsorption but may also affect any part of the body including the heart, lungs, brain, joints, and eyes.

It causes weight loss, an incomplete breakdown of carbohydrates or fats, and malfunctions of the immune system. It is caused by the bacterium *Tropheryma whipplei*, (now known to have one of the smallest genomes of known bacteria) was first described by G H Whipple in 1907. Symptoms include intestinal bleeding, abdominal pain, fatigue, and weight loss. Arthritis and fever often occur several years before intestinal symptoms develop.

Whipple's disease occurs most commonly in middle-aged white men in North America and Europe. The disease is treated with antibiotics, with treatment lasting for one to two years. Treatment lasting less than a year has an approximate relapse rate of 40%.

Treatment, as with other **malabsorption conditions,** in order to help compensate for the vitamins and minerals the body cannot absorb on its own may include:

- extra iron for blood quality as 'iron-deficiency anaemia' is a likely consequence of malabsorption;
- folic acid, as deficiency of this vitamin leads to impaired cell division and it is best derived from fresh vegetables;
- vitamin D for intestinal absorption of calcium, best source is herrings and mackerel; and
- magnesium, which works with calcium in maintaining bone density and nerve and muscle impulses. The lack of magnesium is strongly associated with heart disease, the best source is wheat-germ.

As noted with coeliac disease and Whipple's disease, but especially **with the majority of alimentary canal disorders, the ability of the body to adequately absorb nutrients into the bloodstream is compromised,** often very seriously.

Gastrointestinal malabsorption syndrome is when there is a failure to absorb nutrients as fully as normal. As we have seen, this may be caused by abnormality of the gut wall, failure to produce enzymes and bile to aid digestion, abnormalities of the flora of the gut, or simply a poor diet. In malabsorption syndrome the absorption of essential nutrients is so poor that signs of malnutrition result.

The now familiar symptoms are likely to be present: weakness, weight loss, anaemia, diarrhoea, steatorroea (excessive amount of fat in the stool), abdominal distention with cramps, bloating and gas due to impaired water and carbohydrate absorption, fluid retention (oedema) due to decreased protein absorption as well as muscle wasting, muscle cramping due to decreased absorption of vitamin D, calcium, and magnesium, and peri-anal (around the anus) skin burning, itching, or soreness due to frequent loose stools. Irregular heart rhythms may also result from inadequate levels of potassium and other electrolytes (groups of atoms that conduct electricity). Blood-clotting disorders may occur due to a vitamin K deficiency. Children with malabsorption syndrome often fail to grow and thrive.

Fluid and nutrient monitoring and replacement is essential for any individual with malabsorption syndrome. Hospitalization may be required when severe fluid and electrolyte imbalances occur. In order to further assist the Patient, a consultation with a dietician or nutritional therapist is recommended in order to provide advice about healthy eating and meal planning. The diet needs to be rich in carbohydrates, proteins, fats, minerals, and vitamins and supplements may be taken to provide bulk.

Avoid red meat and dairy products because they stimulate mucous production. The saturated fats found in beef and pork (as well as hydrogenated fats such as margarine) will be harmful as they clog the liver, thus slowing metabolism and inhibiting the absorption of nutrients.

The Patient should be encouraged to eat several small, but frequent, meals throughout the day, avoiding foods that may cause diarrhoea (for example, food with strong spices). The diet should also aim at cleansing and healing the colon. Therefore, a monthly fast may be considered helpful.

In medicine a 'contraindication' (contra literally means against) is a condition or factor that increases the risks involved in using a specific drug, carrying out a medical procedure, or engaging in a particular activity. In other words, the Patient has a symptom/s that makes a particular treatment or therapy inadvisable.

A contraindication may be absolute or relative. For example, in colon hydrotherapy an absolute contraindication would be cancer of the colon. A relative contraindication could be ulcerative colitis (here it would be essential to consider the Patient's frequency to the toilet, whether they are passing blood, whether when feeling their tummy there is any pain and so on).

The wise Practitioner will always be cautious when considering symptoms whether they be contraindicated or indicated. If uncertain about any symptom picture then the first decision must be to ensure the Patient consults with their doctor prior to the commencement of any treatment. Never disregard professional medical advice or delay in seeking it as necessary.

By considering the symptom picture of contraindicated conditions discussed below it becomes clear that an already weakened body is best supported by avoiding any increase of potential pressure and strain upon it that could result from colon hydrotherapy. Always recognise that each person, their symptom condition, and history, is unique. Therefore, if there are ever any questions about the appropriateness of treatment then, as recommended, consult with other professionals. Seeking and exploring a second opinion is always sensible and a sign of being a responsible and professional Practitioner. There is potentially always some risk involved no matter how miniscule. Do not open your practice, or commence your profession as a Practitioner, if you are unprepared or unwilling to assume the risk. It remains the Practitioner's duty, in conjunction with the Patient, is to administer, as far as is possible the safest care at all times.

The Contraindications of Colon Hydrotherapy Treatment. Diseases and Conditions of the Large Intestine, the Liver, The Cardio-Vascular System, and the Kidneys.

The core contraindications of colon hydrotherapy are as follows: cancer of the rectum or bowel; fissures; fistulas; severe haemorrhoids; bowel perforation; recent colon or rectal surgery; gastrointestinal bleeding; cirrhosis of the liver; severe gall stones; high and low blood pressure; aneurism; congestive heart disease; severe anaemia; kidney failure; abdominal hernia; recent scar tissue; a history of steroid use; pregnancy; and uncontrolled diabetes.

CONTRAINDICATIONS DISCUSSED

Diseases and Conditions of the Large Intestine

Cancer of the rectum or bowel is potentially deadly because of its location, hidden away out of sight, in the bowel inside the abdomen, and it often does not cause symptoms until it has had plenty of time to grow and spread. A UK study found that one person in 10, of persons over 45 years of age, with rectal bleeding either had bowel cancer or potentially pre-malignant polyps (Du Toit J, 2006). Fortunately, if the cancer is discovered and treated early enough the cure rate is 90%. The problem is less than 40% are detected early. It is important for people to see a doctor early and to be screened as a precaution for bowel cancer especially if there are any symptoms, particularly bleeding from the back passage or any sign of blood after a bowel motion (often noticed on toilet paper). Colorectal cancer is more common in older people and is rare under the age of forty but the risk increases as a person becomes older.

Fissures are a groove or cleft caused in the skin or mucous membrane by disease. An anal fissure is a break in the lining of the bowel, usually causing pain during bowel movements, and sometimes causing bleeding. Anal fissures usually occur as a consequence of constipation or sometimes diarrhoea.

Fistulas are an abnormal connection of tissue between two organs caused by infection or injury. An anal fistula may develop after an abscess in the rectum has burst creating an opening between the anal canal and the surface of the skin. During the time of the infection the tissues sometimes stick together. If they heal that way a fistula forms.

Another example would be when diverticulitis-related infection spreads outside the colon and the colon's tissue may stick to nearby tissue. The organs usually involved are the bladder, small intestine, and the skin. The most common type of fistula occurs between the bladder and the colon. This type of fistula can result in a severe infection of the urinary tract. Surgery can correct.

Severe haemorrhoids are enlarged, bulging blood vessels in and about the anus and lower rectum. Painless bleeding and protrusion during bowel movements are the most common symptoms. However an internal haemorrhoid can cause severe pain if it is completely prolapsed, that is, protruding from the anal opening. Severe haemorrhoids may require special treatment including surgery (haemorrhoidectomy) and is necessary when clots repeatedly form in external haemorrhoids or when there is persistent bleeding. Eliminating excessive straining reduces pressure on haemorrhoids and helps prevent them from protruding.

A sitz bath, sitting in plain warm water for about 10 minutes, can also provide relief when symptoms are milder. Mild symptoms can also be relieved by increasing fibre (fruit and vegetables) and fluids in the diet. There is no relationship between haemorrhoids and cancer. However, the symptoms, particularly bleeding, are similar to colorectal cancer and other diseases of the digestive tract. The colon hydrotherapist has to be rigorous in considering the mechanical effect of the speculum, water stretching the abdominal cavity, and the risk of excessive bleeding.

Bowel Perforation. Where there is a history of **bowel perforation** colon hydrotherapy must be avoided. A perforated bowel is a medical emergency in which a hole in the bowel opens to allow its contents to empty into the rest of the abdominal cavity. The result is sepsis (the putrefactive destruction of tissues by disease causing bacteria or their toxins) or blood poisoning which if not treated can cause almost immediate death. Symptoms include high fever and nausea. Intestinal blockage can cause a perforated bowel. Patients who have had a perforated bowel will require consistent follow-up and treatment for underlying conditions that may have caused the perforation.

Recent colon or rectal surgery. This usually means cancer is in a part of the bowel and involves taking out a sheet of body tissue called the mesentery, which surround the bowel and rectum. Radiotherapy can be used before surgery to shrink the cancer; after surgery to kill any cancer cells left behind, or to shrink any tumour that may be left. Also surgery is used to treat ulcerative colitis. The prognosis (an estimate of how well the person will remain in the future, often expressed in five-year survival rates) depends upon how advanced the cancer is when treated. Research shows that 88% of Patients with cancer localised within the bowel survive for more than five years plus; 70% of Patients where the cancer has penetrated the bowel wall survive more than five years plus, when the cancer involves the lymph nodes only around 43% survive five years or more. (Fact File Health Library, 2005).

Gastrointestinal (GI) bleeding describes a haemorrhage in the GI tract, from the pharynx to the rectum. The degree of bleeding can range from the nearly undetectable blood to acute and life-threatening bleeding. **Upper GI bleeding**, which is characterized by vomiting up blood (haematemesis) is from a site between the pharynx and the ligament of Treitz (the point where the duodenum connects the stomach to the jejunum. The ligament of Treitz is a supporting band of peritoneum and muscle fibres).

The upper GI tract, also termed the proximal colon, includes the caecum, appendix, ascending colon, hepatic flexure, transverse colon, and the splenic flexure. Lower GI bleeding is indicated by blood being passed through the rectum especially when there is an absence of haematemesis, (the act of vomiting blood). Lower GI tract bleeding, includes the descending colon, sigmoid colon passing blood, and rectum.

Diseases and Conditions of the Liver

Cirrhosis damages the liver permanently and is often caused by drinking too much alcohol. (Cirrhosis is also caused by hepatitis C infection). Symptoms can take years to develop and gradually the function of the liver deteriorates. (Primary biliary cirrhosis is when the bile ducts are attacked by the body's own immune system. Bile deposits in the skin may cause intense itching). Scar tissue replaces normal tissue blocking the flow of blood through the liver. When the liver loses its ability to make the protein albumin water accumulates in the legs (oedema) and abdomen (ascites).

Severe gall stones. Gall is an old-fashioned word for bile, and bile is made in the liver. Gall stones most frequently contain cholesterol and if stuck in the narrow neck of the gall bladder can cause severe pain: biliary colic. (Usually a continuous pain but may also come in waves, found in the middle or just under the ribs on the right-hand side of the body). Gall stones may also cause inflammation of the wall of the gall bladder, jaundice, and pancreatitis. The best test for gall stones is ultrasound.

Diseases and Conditions of the Cardiovascular System

The root cause of most cardiovascular disease is the build up of a fatty deposit within the inside lining of the arteries (artheroma). Cardiovascular diseases are diseases of the heart (cardiac muscle) and the blood vessels (vasculators). Colon hydrotherapists are advised to always take blood pressure readings for first treatments and subsequently monitor.

High and low blood pressure, often referred to, respectively, as hypertension and hypotension. High blood pressure means high pressure (tension) in the arteries. Normal blood pressure is below 120/80, 139/89 is called 'pre-tension', and blood pressure of 140/90 or above is considered high. Uncomplicated high blood pressure usually occurs without symptoms, labelled the silent killer. Actual symptoms include dizziness, blurred vision, and shortness of breath. Severe high blood pressure may cause kidney failure, nausea, heart failure, and stroke. Unlike high blood pressure, low blood pressure is defined by signs and symptoms of the low blood flow and not by a specific blood pressure number.

Some Patients may have a blood pressure reading of 90/50 with no symptoms of low blood pressure. Others who have high blood pressure may develop symptoms of low blood pressure if their blood pressure drops to 100/60. Low blood pressure is a problem when the blood pressure is insufficient to deliver enough blood to the organs of the body. Going from sitting to standing often brings out symptoms of low blood pressure. This occurs because standing causes blood to 'settle' in the veins of the lower body and can lower the blood pressure. If already low, standing can make the low blood pressure worse to the point of causing dizziness or fainting.

Taking the Patient's blood pressure is strongly recommended not only because of the contraindications, but because of its value as an indicator of wider physiological performance and indications. The term 'blood pressure' generally refers to arterial pressure. (That is, pressure in the larger arteries, taking blood away from the heart). Many modern vascular pressure devices, no longer use mercury. Nevertheless, vascular pressure values are still universally reported in millimetres of mercury (mmHg).

In order to obtain an accurate reading it is best that the Patient should not smoke, drink caffeine containing drinks, or engage in strenuous exercise for 30 minutes before taking the reading. For five minutes before the test the Patient should be sitting upright in a chair with their feet flat on the floor and without any limbs crossed. The arm should be relaxed and kept at heart level during the reading. The blood pressure cuff should always be against the skin as readings taken over a sleeve are less accurate. A full bladder may have a small effect on the blood pressure readings so if the urge to urinate exists the Patient should be encouraged to go before the reading.

Practitioners need to acknowledge that an **aneurysm** (a balloon-like swelling in the wall of an artery) is also a contraindication. An aortic aneurysm most frequently occurs in the abdominal aorta, below the level of the renal arteries. Beyond a certain size it is prone to rupture, thus presenting an acute surgical emergency.

Congestive heart disease (heart failure) is a condition that can result from any structural or functional cardiac disorder that impairs the ability of the heart to fill with or pump a sufficient amount of blood through the body. This condition can affect many organs. For example, kidney function may be diminished causing the retention of more fluid in the body; the lungs can become congested with fluid; fluid may likewise accumulate in the liver impairing the elimination of toxins; moreover, intestines may become less efficient at absorbing nutrients.

Congestive heart failure will affect virtually every organ over time. A thorough Patient history may disclose the presence of one or more related symptoms being present, particularly fatigue, oedema, and shortness of breath, (especially at night when the Patient may describe awakening and gasping for air). Due to a lack of a universally agreed definition heart disease is often undiagnosed, and it is the leading cause of hospitalization in people older than 65.

Severe anaemia. Red blood cells contain a substance called haemoglobin. Haemoglobin binds to oxygen and takes oxygen from the lungs to every part of the body. To constantly make red blood cells and haemoglobin the body needs healthy bone marrow and nutrients such as iron and vitamins (B12). Anaemia means having fewer red blood cells than normal, or, having less haemoglobin than normal in each red cell. Due to the reduced oxygen level common symptoms include: tiredness, lethargy, feeling faint, poor concentration, general malaise, and easily becoming breathless (dyspnoea). In more severe cases headaches, palpitations, altered taste, and ringing in the ears may be reported. Severe anaemia prompts the body to compensate by increasing output leading to palpitations, sweatiness, and heart failure.

Diseases and Conditions of the Kidney

Kidney failure is a serious disease having a major impact of life and can be fatal. The body retains fluid, blood pressure rises, harmful wastes build up in the body, and the body fails to make enough red blood cells. The waste products urea and creatinine cause tiredness, loss of appetite, and vomiting.

Abdominal hernia is usually noticed as a lump in the groin or the umbilical region. It may be either painless or painful. It appears when a portion of the tissues that line the abdominal cavity (peritoneum) breaks through a weakened area of the abdominal wall. This can be extremely dangerous if a piece of the intestine becomes trapped (strangulated) inside. This can lead to gangrenous (dead) bowel in as little as six hours. Activities that increase abdominal pressure may cause the hernia to increase in size.

Contraindications Concerning Other Conditions

Scar tissue, (from injury or operation, if less than two month since received). A scar is a mark left in the skin (or organ) by the healing of a wound, is the replacement of tissue by connective tissue made up of collagen. (Collagen is an important body protein that is the basic matrix of connective tissue, bone, cartilage, and skin found in fish, wheat-germ, vegetables, and fruit). Complications, such as infections, that impede healing can also increase the amount of scar tissue. Too much tension on a healing wound can also increase scar formation. Tension, exercise, and stretching and can prolong the inflammation and healing process.

History of steroid use (oral use over one year). Steroid use is valuable for a range of conditions and can be life saving. They have potent anti-inflammatory properties. However, side effects can occur especially with long-term use. Changes in sugar levels can occur; the immune system can become suppressed leaving the body susceptible to infection; bone texture can change due to calcium loss; the skin can become thin; can cause stomach ulcers; other medication may be needed if fluid builds up or there is any loss of the mineral potassium. Potassium is one of the main blood minerals, called electrolytes. The other main minerals are sodium and chloride. All are essential for both cellular and electrical function. (It is the kidneys that are the main regulators of the body's potassium).

Pregnancy. Colon hydrotherapy is essentially a natural process and although there is virtually no danger there is always some risk. Moreover, because of the very special nature of pregnancy and the particular risks associated with possible miscarriage and other complications caution is always advised. Although it would be difficult to legally demonstrate that colon hydrotherapy was the cause of a miscarriage, it is clinically wise to wait until several months after the birth of the child when the mother is fully recovered. Some colon hydrotherapists do give treatments but avoid the first three months and final month. Clearly, it would be sensible to refrain treatment during complicated pregnancies.

However, there is some evidence to show that inflammatory bowel disease doubles the risk of pregnancy complications, that is: premature birth and children born below normal weight. Moreover the rate of congenital birth defects in babies born to mothers with the disorders is more than twice as high. (St Mary's Hospital, London, BBC News, Health, 2006). Remember also that a further concern to be mindful of is that the risk of complications increases with the age of the woman.

Uncontrolled diabetes. Type 2 diabetes is a condition that occurs when the pancreas fails to produce enough insulin or the body's cells stop responding to the insulin that is produced. In either case, glucose in the blood cannot be absorbed or used by the cells of the body. It is a complex disorder that has many possible indicators. For example: unexplained weight loss, excessive hunger, thirst, frequent urination, dehydration, leg pain when walking, fatigue, dizziness, and itching.

There are two main types of diabetes. Type 1 is called insulin-dependent diabetes because people who develop it need to have insulin injections at least once a day. (Also called juvenile diabetes as it commonly begins in childhood or adolescence). The more common form is type 2, and can often be controlled with diet and oral medication (often with one of the drugs from the group known as statins). Type 2 is sometimes called adult/age-onset diabetes and occurs most often in people over 50 years of age. The consequences of uncontrolled type 2 diabetes are as serious as those caused by type 1.

Note: the blood-sugar levels seen in diabetes increase the progression of atherosclerosis and cardiovascular disease. Colon hydrotherapy may affect blood-sugar levels due to absorption of additional water. Moreover, Patients who are diabetic are more susceptible to infection if the disease is inadequately controlled. High levels of blood glucose (hyperglycaemia) are also toxic. (See section on Diet and Nutrition, and Table 1, The Glycaemic Index).

Note: foods with a low glycaemic index, which release sugar more slowly into the bloodstream, appear to play a major role in helping Patients with diabetes control their disease. It is recommended to keep glucose in the treatment room in case a Patient feels faint or dizzy.

Given all of the foregoing section it is clear that the skilled Practitioner will need to always be mindful, and take full account of, the Patient's medical history, current symptoms, and potential for having contraindicative problems. The task requires the Practitioner to proceed with insight and caution. It is believed that in the hands of a qualified and skilled Practitioner colon hydrotherapy is unlikely to cause harm whatever the problem may be. (Collings J, 1996).

Nevertheless, in the interests of Patient care and safety, and the avoidance of any unforeseen and unexpected consequences, it is imperative that patient's with conditions that are contraindicative are declined treatment, or referred immediately, to the respective Patient's GP for advice and guidance, prior to any consideration of treatment, no matter how tentative that treatment may be. It is only then that the potential for placing the Patient and Practitioner in vulnerable (or liable) positions will be avoided, and safe care maintained.

The Indications for Colon Hydrotherapy Treatment

In the interests of clarity, easier reference, and application, this important section is sub-divided into eight indication groupings. These groupings relate, as far as is possible, the respective indications to their anatomical systems. We know of the complexity of the body and Its physiological systems and that these function within a fully and perfectly integrated whole. Our preference therefore, is to treat the Patient in accordance with naturopathic principles and endeavour to treat them holistically within their symptom profile. In terms of treatment strategies there will be an inter-relationship concerning symptoms and treatment and goals.

It is suggested, that the grouping of indications provides for easier management and understanding of all these concerns, and assists the Practitioner in maintaining both consistency and rigour, and ensures that the Patient's needs remain paramount.

Before we examine in detail the indications for colon hydrotherapy within the proposed **eight separate groupings**, a list of the indications to be explored is provided as follows:

GROUP ONE

The Large Intestine:

Constipation

Diarrhoea

Irritable Bowel Syndrome

Gas

Bloating

Bowel Noises

Belching

Ulcerative Colitis

Intestinal Toxaemia

Ileocaecal Valve Ssyndrome

Preparation for Bowel Investigation

GROUP TWO

Circulation, Venous, and Lymphatic Disorder

Circulation and Venous Function

Lymphatic Disorder

GROUP THREE
Hormonal Disorders and Hypoglycemia

Hormonal Disorders

Hypoglycaemia

GROUP FOUR

Digestive Disorders

Gastritis

Food Allergies

GROUP FIVE

Parasite and Fungal Infection

Parasite infestation or infections

Candida albicans

Cystitis

Halitosis (infection in tooth cavities, gums, and colon-related issues)

GROUP SIX

Skin Disorders

Eczema

Psoriasis

Acne

GROUP SEVEN

Other Chronic Conditions:

Chronic Fatigue Syndrome (CFS)

Myalgic Encephalomylitis (ME)

Asthma

Arthritis

Gout

GROUP EIGHT

Other Relevant Conditions:

Headaches and Migraines

Sleep Disorders

Back pain

INDICATIONS DISCUSSED

GROUP ONE

The Large Intestine:

Constipation is one of the most common digestive complaints.

It varies greatly between people, as each person's bowel movements differ, and it saps the health of millions of people. Remember, **constipation is a symptom not a disease.** Almost everyone experiences constipation at some point in their life and poor diet typically is the cause. Most of the time it is not serious and is a temporary condition. Understanding its causes, prevention, and treatment will provide relief for most people.

Many cases of constipation are caused by a low-fibre diet or dehydration, lack of exercise, or immobility, and may arise as a side effect of medications (especially antidepressants). The symptoms are infrequent bowel movements, the passage of hard stools, and difficulty in passing stools. During physical examination, **scybala** (manually detectable lumps of stool) may be detected on palpation of the abdomen. Constipation is more common in children and older people and affects women more than men. One in 200 women have severe, continuous constipation and it is most common before a period and in pregnancy. (NHS, 2007).

Normal bowel movements vary between people. Some go more than once a day; others may go every two or three days. Variations in your normal daily routines, like taking a break from work, going on holiday, going on a training course, can result in fewer visits to the toilet. Constipation is infrequent bowel movement (and can alternate with diarrhoea). Constipation is when a person has difficulty defecating, when it be comes necessary to strain. This can be painful and cause bleeding. When stools are very small the muscles around the anus are unable to grip them properly in order to eliminate them. Stools dry up and go back into the colon, shrink more, and block the passage, meaning constipation will continue, often causing an infrequent urge to void. Constipation is present when there is also the sensation of incomplete bowel evacuation.

Ideally bowel movement should be twice a day, one for each main meal, of loose consistency (where the stools break in water) and of an inoffensive odour. An adequate transit time per meal is considered to be between 12 to 24 hours. (See Figure 2). This can be tested by eating non-digestible foods such as whole peanuts, corn on the cob, or tomato skin. Evidence of transit time can also be measured by consuming seeds such as linseed, sunflower, and pumpkin seeds. Simply measure the time it takes from consumption and the time these appear in your stools.

Although many people use **laxatives** (or **purgatives)**, laxatives are not the answer to constipation. These compounds or drugs, taken to induce bowel movements, can also cause diarrhoea and significant flatulence, and are often abused by people. Laxative abuse is potentially serious. **Laxative use** can cause **side effects** such as: inadequate bowel flora, irritated mucosa of the colon, food allergies, kidney disease, pancreatitis, mineral deficiencies, depression, worse constipation, and IBS. The routine non-medical use of laxatives is to be discouraged as they can result in bowel action becoming dependent upon their use.

Temporary relief from constipation may be achieved by having figs and prunes with breakfast. Also the seeds and husks of *psyllium/* linseeds are a safe and effective remedy. In order to stimulate bowel movement drink hot water with fresh lemon juice. Lemons are especially tonic and act as cleansers when toxicity exists in the liver, kidneys, bowels, lungs, and skin.

The symptoms of constipation vary between people. They include:

Stomach ache and cramps

Feeling bloated and feeling sick

Not feeling empty, or a sense of feeling full

Haemorrhoids

Headache

Back ache

Loss of appetite

Furred tongue, bad breath

Fatigue/low energy

Depression

Skin indications

Mucous build-up (nasal passages)

Constipation is caused when motility is slow and the colon then absorbs too much water. Alternatively, if the colon's muscle contractions are slow, or sluggish, thus again, causing the stool to move through the colon too slowly. Moreover, people who ignore or frequently delay the urge to have a bowel movement (often because of stress, and/or because they are too busy, or do not wish to interrupt what they are doing) may eventually stop feeling the need for bowel movement. This functional constipation means the bowel is likely to be healthy but not working properly and can affect the whole body.

Although treatment (and prevention) will depend upon cause, severity, duration, and lifestyle, measures to be taken to avoid constipation and prevent recurrence will include the following matters.

Constipation: Suggestions for Discussion with the Patient as part of Developing the Treatment Plan

- Lifestyle and adjustments concerning the eating of a well-balanced, high-fibre diet that includes pulses, beans, whole grains, fresh fruit (plums, figs, kiwi fruit, or pear before breakfast) and vegetables. Include discussing the benefits of bulking agents, for example: linseeds, *psyllium* husks, oat bran. Note: raisins soaked in water, or four or five dried figs soaked in water over-night will also help.

- Drinking plenty of water (filtered) and avoiding caffeine, alcohol, and fizzy drinks.

- Exercising, as appropriate for the respective Patient, regularly,

114

and encouraging use of the 'complete breath' (See section Five Systems of Elimination, the Lungs).

- Eating breakfast comfortably. Setting aside time for undisturbed visits to the toilet, (understanding that normal bowel habits vary but seek advice if believed to be significant).

- Discuss 'potty training' and not ignoring the urge to have a bowel movement and use 'squatting' position with foot stool for assistance.

- The benefits of avoiding (or reducing) the intake of processed foods such as cheese, cakes/biscuits, and white bread.

- It may be appropriate to consider herbal laxatives (for example, Cascara compound, herbal laxative tea) for the short term (not if pregnant), and review use after six weeks.

- Also consider digestive enzyme supplements (some products also contain bile and liver herbs which help lubricate the bowel).

- Use *acidophilus* to restore bowel flora.

Diarrhoea is the passing of frequent, watery stools. It is a symptom that can be acute or chronic. Acute diarrhoea is usually caused by a viral or a bacterial infection and affects almost everyone from time to time. It usually clears up in a couple of days, but does carry the risk of dehydration. Chronic diarrhoea (lasting more than two weeks in an adult) may be because of more serious disorders and should always be investigated by the Patient's doctor.

Symptoms of Diarrhoea may include:

Cramp-like stomach pains

Nausea and vomiting

Fever

Headache

Loss of appetite

Diarrhoea occurs when the lining of the small or large intestine is irritated. This leads to increased water being passed to the stools. Besides viruses or bacteria being a cause, short-term causes may also include: emotional upset or anxiety, alcohol, coffee, side effects of medicine, or allergy. Long-term conditions that cause chronic diarrhoea and discussed above include: ulcerative colitis, Crohn's disease, IBS, and food intolerance.

If suffering from acute diarrhoea avoid dehydration by drinking lots of water. The Patient is more likely to become dehydrated if they are also vomiting. (Rehydration drinks are available and these sachets provide the correct balance of water, salts, and sugar. They do not help cure the diarrhoea but help prevent dehydration). Antidiarrhoea medicines can relieve the symptoms of severe diarrhoea but can also cause constipation. Following a period of calm, eat as soon as your body tells you it is likely to be safe to do so. Chew foods well, foods high in carbohydrates (brown bread, rice, potatoes) and continue drinking lots of water. Avoid milk and other dairy products, raw vegetables, and fruit until improvement. Always maintain high standards of hygiene.

Note: bowel **incontinence** is the loss of bowel control resulting in the involuntary passage of stool. The most common cause, ironically, is constipation, which causes the muscles of the anus (and intestines) to stretch and weaken. The weakened muscles will prevent the rectum from closing tightly thus resulting in leakage. The nerves of anus and rectum also become less responsive to the presence of stool. To hold stool and maintain continence requires the normal function of the bowel and the nervous system. Additionally the person must posses the physical and psychological ability to recognize and appropriately respond to the urge to defecate. Treatment begins with identifying the cause.

Diarrhoea: Suggestions for Discussion with the Patient as

Part of Developing the Treatment Plan.

- Ensure the Patient discusses symptom/s with GP.

- The treatment of diarrhoea will be as for constipation if symptom picture indicates alternating symptoms.

- It is important to increase water intake.

- Discuss avoiding spicy foods, potential sources of allergy (dairy, gluten, wheat, citrus), alcohol, coffee, and refer to diet for constipation but avoid excessive quantities of raw food.

- Discuss stress-related issue and further life-style matters, which may be contributing to the problem.

- Supplements for consideration include: *psyllium* husk, aloe vera, which are soothing, a mineral supplement in order to compensate for loss. Carrot soup is effective and replenishes sodium, potassium, phosphorus, calcium, and magnesium. Will help allay intestinal inflammation and check growth of harmful bacteria. Mint tea is also beneficial.

- Suggest *acidophilus* to restore bowel flora.

Irritable Bowel Syndrome. IBS is a syndrome, given that it is not a defined disease. The picture or syndrome most commonly includes constipation, diarrhoea, bloating (day or night), with abdominal pain being the most common symptom. The pain may be mild or severe and may be made either better or worse by opening the bowels, passing wind, or eating. Other symptoms, although not comprehensive, are headaches; passing urine more frequently; fatigue and tiredness; sleep disturbance; loss of appetite; nausea; anxiety and stress; with depressive symptoms in about a third of Patients. IBS is the most common condition seen by gastroenterologists. **(Gastroenterology is the study of GI disease, in any part of the digestive tract, also the liver, biliary tract, and pancreas).**

The first symptoms are usually experienced between the ages of 15 and 40 and IBS is more common in women. It is estimated that as many as one in five adults in the UK have IBS at any one time! IBS is often associated with hormonal or emotional factors like anxiety, depression, or stress indicating a complex interaction between psychological and physical factors. As a disorder of the digestive system can affect the system, anywhere from the mouth to the anus, this accounts for the diversity of symptoms seen in IBS.

It is unknown what causes IBS, although half of people with IBS date the start of their symptoms to a major life event (for example, bereavement, or change of job). Ten to 20% date their symptoms to an acute bout of gastroenteritis (inflammation of the stomach that causes vomiting and diarrhoea). For the remainder, the trigger factor/s remains unidentified. Symptoms can change over time. It is a **functional disorder** meaning that the way the bowel works is affected but medical tests find no physical abnormalities.

Diagnosis is made on the basis of typical symptoms. There is no single blood test, X-ray, or scan that will diagnose IBS and as the cause is unknown it is not possible to reliably prevent symptoms. IBS usually occurs periodically throughout life. The symptoms can improve, get worse, or disappear for years. **Note: up to 60% of people defined with the syndrome have psychological symptoms such as anxiety and depression.** (See section on 'Emotions and Feelings').

In addition to colon hydrotherapy, the treatment plan for most Patients, with IBS will be the use of self-help methods aimed at improving symptoms.

Irritable Bowel Syndrome: Suggestions for Discussion with the Patient as Part of Developing the Treatment Plan

- The value of drinking lots of water. For people with constipation this helps the fibre to work; for people with diarrhoea it replaces lost fluid (preferably 2l a day). Also essential to have an hydrated system for optimum health. Consider the possibility of *Candida* or parasites being the cause.

- The gradual introduction of a high-fibre diet. Fibre-rich foods help stabilise the symptoms. Avoid irritants or triggers like coffee, milk, and strong spicy foods (that cause wind) which are frequent offenders. Alcohol intake and carbonated drinks are likely to worsen symptoms. Eliminate milk and dairy products and have a food intolerance test. (It is recognised that not everyone has milk intolerance and that problems may easily be associated with other food, Nevertheless, milk intolerance is extremely common which is why a food allergy test is recommended).

- Suggest keeping a diary of which foods seem to be the cause of upset.

- Avoiding large meals but eating regularly to assist bowel habit, can improve digestion and also reduce stress.

- Consider complementary treatments alongside colon hydrotherapy such as: heat treatments, detoxification regimes, relaxation techniques, and massage, as a way of improving general health status.

- Rest as much as possible but combine with the 'complete breath' (that is, breathing as if into the tummy allowing the tummy to rise and then hold the breath for a second and take a second breath without exhaling the first up into the lungs and pulling the breath as if up into the collar bones. Then exhaling, emptying from the top downward). When improvement noticed increase exercise.

- Discuss digestive enzymes, the entire system depends upon enzymatic action and supplementation is likely to be necessary.

- *Acidophilus* to restore bowel flora.

Gas, Bloating, Bowel Noises, and Belching. Complaints from Patients about having too much gas, wind, flatulence, belching, breaking wind, and feeling bloated are very common. Every day a normal individual passes wind through the back passage, intestinal gas known as **flatus**, 15 times (ranging between three and 40

119

times), depending upon diet. High-fibre diets produce more wind although it is possible to avoid those foods which produce greater amounts of gas and maintain high-fibre intake. Reduce foods which cannot be digested in the small intestines (containing carbohydrates called oligosaccharide) but are food to bacteria in the colon. For example, cabbage, sprouts, onions, and seeds such as fennel and sunflower.

Moreover, some people have difficulty in digesting lactose, the sugar in cow's milk. As a result, the lactose is fermented by the colon bacteria thus producing large amounts of carbon dioxide and hydrogen. Flatus is composed partly of swallowed air and partly of gas produced by bacterial fermentation of intestinal contents. Flatus consists mainly of five gases: nitrogen, oxygen, carbon dioxide, hydrogen, and methane.

Remember, the small intestine is where the food we eat is digested and absorbed. The residues, such as dietary fibre and some carbohydrates, pass on to the bowel. The colon acts as a gas works. It contains a huge population of many different kinds of bacteria that are essential to good health and it is these that ferment the residues delivered from the small intestines, producing large volumes of gas. Most of these gases are absorbed into the blood stream and eventually excreted in the breath. The rest is passed as flatus. Smelly wind is caused by substances like indoles, skatoles, and hydrogen sulphide that are again produced by bacterial fermentation in the colon.

Bloating is associated with abdominal distension. This is usually due to relaxation of the abdominal muscles in an unconscious attempt to relieve discomfort. The distension usually disappears on lying flat or on contracting the abdominal muscles. A high-fibre diet may relieve bloating because fibre absorbs water in the gut and gently distends it, helping to prevent the uncoordinated contractions that are partly responsible for bloating. Some people find charcoal to be helpful. Colon hydrotherapy will certainly help the conditions that give rise to bloating.

Bowel noises (borborygmi) are produced when the liquid and gases of the intestines are shuffled backwards and forwards by vigorous contraction of the gut. Can be caused by hunger, or anxiety, is common with IBS, or with diseases of the intestine like Crohn's disease, or to overcome obstruction. Be mindful of any associated symptoms, such as severe abdominal pain, which need to be reported to the Patient's doctor.

Belching or burping is usually an involuntary expulsion of wind by the stomach when it becomes distended from an excess of swallowed air. Eating rapidly, gulping food and drink, smoking, wearing loose dentures all promote air swallowing. Some people develop aerophagy (repetitive burping) because of discomfort in the chest.

Gas, Bloating, Bowel Noise, and Belching: Suggestions for Discussion with the Patient as Part of Developing the Treatment Plan

- Life-style issues associated with a diet high in sugars and processed food, coffee, alcohol, and poor nutrition.

- Discuss need to respond to the need to go to the toilet, using the squatting posture to eliminate wind and stool.

- Need to avoid drinking with meals, chew food thoroughly, and avoid too much food, and spicy food.

- Consider parasite, liver, and kidney cleanse.

- Digestive enzymes will be important as symptom group relate to digestion.

- Discuss need for exercise, relaxation, and deep breathing.

Ulcerative Colitis is a chronic, relapsing condition and the severity of symptoms and how frequently they occur will vary from Patient to Patient. Between flare-ups of the symptoms the inflamed areas of colon and rectum heal. About half of people with ulcerative colitis have mild and infrequent symptoms. The other half will have frequent flare-ups with moderate to severe symptoms.

With the flare-up, symptoms will include: mild to severe diarrhoea that may be mixed with mucous, blood, or pus. An urgency to get to the toilet is common; a feeling of wanting to get to the toilet (tenesmus) but with nothing to pass is also common. As water is not absorbed so well in the inflamed colon then diarrhoea will be watery. Alternatively, the Patient may have normal stools rather than diarrhoea and may even become constipated accompanied with a frequent feeling of wanting to go to the toilet. Pain when passing stools is likely to occur, also cramp like pains in the abdomen. Remember, with flare-ups Patient's may also be feeling generally unwell, tired, feeling sick, showing weight loss, be feverish, and anaemia may develop. Note: clearly convey the message to all Patients that whatever the condition **all food must be chewed slowly and thoroughly, before swallowing.**

Ulcerative Colitis: Suggestions for Discussion with the Patient as Part of Developing the Treatment Plan

- Review ways of improving digestion, and as noted chew food thoroughly, avoid large meals, and eating late in the evening. Eliminate coffee and all other sources of caffeine. Food allergies, consumption of sugar and refined foods; parasites/Candida to be addressed.

- Reduce inflammation with aloe vera. Slippery elm tea. Garlic, which is alkaline, is an effective cleanser and aids digestion. During flare-ups, avoid raw fruits and vegetables, seeds, and nuts.

- Chlorophyll supplement to promote healing.

- Vitamin B12 supplement may be necessary. Fresh beetroot juice will be helpful for its high iron content and its potassium, phosphorous, calcium, iodine, copper, vitamins, and carbohydrate properties.

- A further consideration could be a juice fast for up to five days (include raw cabbage juice and carrot juice). Avoid citrus juices. After the fast, adopt a diet of small frequent meals of steamed vegetables, rice, ripe fruit like banana and seeds and grains. Raw vegetables to be added gradually after two weeks and after problems have subsided.

- Need to avoid constipation.

- *Acidophilus* to restore bowel flora

Intestinal Toxaemia. (Also see, The Principles of Natural Therapeutics , Diseases of the Bowel, and Cleansing and Detoxification Sections).

"Every physician should realise that the intestinal toxaemias are the most important primary and contributing causes of many disorders and diseases of the human body" (Bassler A, 1933).

The GI tract must digest and process food, selectively absorb essential nutrients, and biochemicals and eliminate toxic, allergenic, and inflammatory compounds and poisons.

As noted in the Royal Society of Medicine Report 1913, the recorded 36 poisons of alimentary intestinal toxaemia, although not necessarily the sole course of all the various symptoms and disorders discussed, are serious contributors. It is also true that since that time we consume more processed foods, have removed more nutrients from our food, increased the chemical fertilizers and insecticides used in the production of crops and harvests, created poorer soils, and regularly feed antibiotics and growth hormones to animals, thus adding significantly more toxicity for our GI tract to deal with.

The **microflora** in the small and large intestines must be in balance to ensure the health and proper functioning of the intestinal mucosa. Imbalances can alter the immunological and mechanical integrity of the mucosa thus permitting the absorption of toxins (leaky gut). The liver must detoxify the body by also removing endogenous (derived from within the body) waste products, the end-products of metabolism, and the toxic chemicals that have been ingested, inhaled, and absorbed through the skin.

'The colon is a sewage system but by neglect and abuse it becomes a cesspool. When it is clean and normal we are well and happy; let it stagnate and it will distil the poisons of decay, fermentation and putrefaction into the blood, poisoning the brain and nervous system so that we become mentally depressed and irritable; it will poison the heart

123

so we are weak and listless; poisons the lungs so that the breath is foul; poisons the digestive organs so that we are distressed and bloated; and poisons the blood so that the skin is sallow and unhealthy. In short, every organ of the body is poisoned and we age prematurely, look and feel old, the joints are stiff and painful, dull eyes and a sluggish brain overtake us; the pleasure of living is gone'. (Newman R, 2007).

Intestinal Toxaemia: Suggestions for Discussion with the Patient as Part of Developing the Treatment Plan.

- The need for regular colon hydrotherapy in order to cleanse the bowel and therefore decrease the production and absorption of toxins. Discuss cleansing and detoxification.

- Include probiotic supplements to promote bowel flora.

- Address matters as outlined for Patients with constipation.

Ileocaecal valve syndrome. The ileocaecal valve is located between the ileum (the last portion of the small intestine) and the caecum, which is the first portion of the large intestine. The ileocaecal valve evolved to be a one-way valve, only opening up to allow the semi-liquid digested food materials and wastes through into the caecum. It also blocks these waste materials from backing up and returning into the small intestine.

The ileocaecal valve syndrome, also known as Konig's syndrome, is a syndrome of mainly abdominal pain in relation to meals, constipation alternating with diarrhoea, tympanites, (distention of the abdomen with air or gas making the abdomen resonant, drum-like on percussion), gurgling sounds (hyper-peristalsis) on auscultation, which is listening with the aid of a stethoscope to sounds produced by the movement of gas, especially in the right iliac fissure and abdominal extension. Furthermore, a dysfunctional ileocaecal valve can result in a combination of other disorders, for example: pain in the right shoulder, right-side pelvic pain, low-back pain, tinnitus, dark circles under the eyes, pain surrounding the heart.

The syndrome is caused by an incomplete obstruction of the small

124

intestine and especially the ileocaecal valve as, for example in Crohn's disease, or in rare cases of cancer of the small intestine. (Franz Konig, 1832 to 1910). Other causes are thought to include: dehydration, emotional upset, eating too quickly and too frequently, under-chewing food, eating hot spicy foods.

Ileocaecal Valve Syndrome: Suggestions for Discussion with Patient as Part of Developing the Treatment Plan

- The need to drink plenty of water in order to assist motility and general metabolism and absorption.

- As with IBS discuss the need to avoid stimulants, sugar, foods containing sugar, also avoid refined carbohydrates and spicy foods.

- The need to chew food well, and to avoid raw foods for a couple of weeks in order to enable the ileocaecal valve to recover. Avoid wheat bran.

- Consider including deep massage when acute, and use hot and cold compresses.

- Consider *Candida* or parasite as possible cause.

- Consider digestive enzymes. (Scottish School of Colon Hydrotherapy, 2007).

Preparation for Bowel Investigation. Patients with varying conditions undergo imaging of the rectum and colon, for example, with sigmoidoscopy and colonoscopy. It is essential for any investigation to be effective and accurate that a clear image of the mucosa is achieved so that pathology that might otherwise be out of view is seen. Preparation is about clearing the colon. Most bowel examinations are undertaken as out-patient procedures and therefore in most cases bowel preparation can be undertaken away from the hospital.

Colon hydrotherapy use can be planned well in advance of examination and can also be used post-barium meal use when undergoing radiography examination of the GI tract, especially as some Patients find it very difficult to expel. To help clear before an investigation (or colon hydrotherapy), Patients may find one tablespoon of Epsom Salt in water useful.

INDICATIONS GROUP TWO

Circulation, Venous and Lymphatic Disorders and Conditions

The primary function of venous circulation is to return blood to the heart, to be pumped to the lungs, to be re-oxygenated and recirculated to the body. As the circulatory system is a closed circuit venous return must equal the flow of blood back into the body via the arteries. The flow varies with activity, temperature, and is largely controlled through selective arterial constrictions.

When aetiological factors (causes of disease) cause a loss of balance of fluid movement it may result in increased interstitial fluid (fluid between the cells) at a systemic level. Diseases of the kidneys and liver may result in generalized oedema. Certain drugs such as steroids, hormone therapies, and some antidepressants, may cause the same. In the case of infection, oedema can be short lived.

Malfunctions in the lymphatic system, damage to the lymph ducts or nodes, prevents the lymphatic vessels from draining away the normal quotient of interstitial fluid. Inadequate flow of the circulatory system can lead to stasis and all the associated affects of stagnation.

Dry skin brushing, particularly the lymph nodes under the breast muscles, and tapping the sternum can also help the lymph system's ability to detoxify. Naturopaths make frequent use of reflex therapy.

Chapman's Reflexes are palpable gangliform contractions located in specific anatomical areas, which can be related to specific organs or glands. In general, Chapman's Reflexes are found in soft tissue at various points along both sides of the sternum, the proximal head of the humerus, distal and proximal clavicle, occipital ridge, clavicle, ribs, scapula, thoracics, lumbar, sacrum, coccyx, pelvis, pubis, fibula, and medial head of the tibia. Chapman's Reflexes is just a term given to these receptor organs because of the osteopath who discovered their diagnostic and therapeutic value in the location and treatment of disease.

Circulation, Venous and Lymphatic Disorders and Conditions: Suggestions for Discussion with the Patient as Part of Developing the Treatment Plan.

- Explore the clear benefits to be gained from colon hydrotherapy treatments. (Some Practitioners also use colon hydrotherapy with decongestive lymphatic drainage techniques, a specialized massage that stimulates lymphatic flow, which has been shown to reduce the incidence of infection, reduce oedema, and promote venous and lymphatic flow).

- Remember that salt causes the body to retain water therefore the avoidance of salty foods may be advised.

- Consider a low-fat diet and increase omega-3 fatty acids, especially essential fatty acids from salmon, sardines, and fortified eggs.

- If appropriate the Patient may be encouraged to exercise as another way of getting rid of excessive fluid and stimulating blood flow.

- Consume alkaline-forming foods. Avoid acid-forming refined foods and animal products as nearly all contain cholesterol and fat.

- Boost the immune system with beta-carotene, found in orange vegetables and sweet potatoes; from vitamin E found in grains and beans; and from vitamin C, which is in many fruits and vegetables.

INDICATIONS GROUP THREE

Hormonal Disorders and Hypoglycaemia:

As stated at the beginning of this section, the body works as a whole system and nothing indicates that more clearly than the endocrine system. The endocrine system is a complex group of **glands** that helps to control reproduction, metabolism, and growth and development, through substances called hormones. **Hormones** have a profound effect on our everyday health and wellbeing. Although present in only minute amounts, hormones act on every cell of the body.

Not only do hormones have their individual effects, but they also interact with each other to produce dramatic influences on the body. Hormones can therefore be defined as chemical messengers. In some instances an organ may have an internal hormonal secretion that enters the blood directly, and an external secretion which leaves it by a duct. The pancreas is an example. The internal secretion of the pancreas, insulin, passes in to the blood, while the pancreatic juice reaches the duodenum via the pancreatic duct.

Important ductless glands are the **thyroid and parathyroid, adrenal, pituitary, thymus, pineal, and Islets of Langerhans in the pancreas, and sex glands.**

The liver and stomach also produce hormones. For example the liver synthesizes and secretes at least three important hormones, **insulin-like growth factor-1 (IGF-1),** which is the immediate stimulus for growth of the body; **angiotensin** which plays a role in maintaining blood pressure; and **thrombopoietin** which stimulates precursor cells in the bone marrow concerning the generation of platelets, essential to blood clotting. Regarding the stomach, over two dozen hormones have been indentified in various parts of the gastrointestinal tract. For example, **gastrin** secreted by cells in the stomach and duodenum that stimulates the secretion of gastric juice and the enzyme pepsin; **secretin** which stimulates the pancreas to secrete bicarbonate into the pancreatic fluid thus neutralizing the acidity of the intestinal contents.

There are **many symptoms associated with hormone imbalance,** for example: depression, hot flushes, heavy or painful periods, low libido, mood swings, poor concentration, decreased strength, erectile dysfunction, sleep disturbances, constipation, IBS, thrush, palpitations, hypoglycaemia, high blood pressure, cystitis, bladder infrequency, hearing loss, and reduced perspiration (Budd M, 2000).

Hormonal Disorders may be reflected in many of the symptoms Patients are worried about. The **adrenal glands** are situated on the upper pole of each kidney and produce three types of steroid hormones, (including adrenalin), which enable the body to respond to the stresses of daily life. Such is secreted into the blood at the onset of danger, anger, excitement, or stress and is responsible for many of the changes that accompany these emotions. These hormones also help to maintain blood-sugar levels and promote a healthy immune system. (Budd, 2000)

Symptoms of adrenal imbalance include: allergies, chemical sensitivities, sugar cravings, sleep disturbances, fatigue, memory loss and unable to turn mind off, high blood-sugar, low immunity, developing colds, poor digestion, and constipation. Disease of the adrenal glands in adult life results in a condition known as Addison's disease. This is characterized byZ low blood pressure, digestive disturbances, and a brown pigmentation of the skin and mucous membrane. There is an excessive loss of sodium from the body and dehydration is common.

Thyroid hormone imbalance leads to hypothyroidism, meaning the body has inadequate levels of the thyroid hormone. (Hyperthyroidism is a less common condition and exists when excess thyroid, for example, bulging eyes are a symptom). The thyroid hormone thyroxine is made from the amino acid tyrosine. The enzyme that converts one into the other is dependent on iodine, zinc, and selenium.

As every cell is affected by thyroid hormones, symptoms of imbalances are often varied and affect multiple body systems. Symptoms include feeling cold, shortness of breath, menstrual irregularities, premenstrual tension, dry skin, decreased sweating, fatigue, low libido, tight sensation and swelling around the neck (goitre), constipation, and weight gain in underactive thyroid, weight loss in overactive thyroid.

The Barnes Axillary Temperature Test provides for testing basal metabolic rates. It was devised and tested by Dr Broda Barnes in the United States. He spent 44 years studying hypothyroidism and published his discoveries in the book: 'Hypothyroidism: The Unsuspected Illness'. As there may be many other causes for the suggested symptoms above, thyroid (hormonal) problems can often be overlooked.

If the Patient has several of the symptoms noted, then nothing is lost by utilizing the Barnes Axillary Test. If the test shows the Patient's temperature to be consistently subnormal then it would be sensible to suggest a blood or urine test. The Axillary Temperature Test for Thyroid Function requires the Patient to undertake the following:

- Before retiring to bed to shake down a thermometer and place it within easy reach of the bed.

- Upon waking, immediately place the thermometer under the armpit for ten minutes. It is essential that the Patient remains still and quiet in order to achieve an accurate reading.

- After 10 minutes read the temperature and record on the chart provided.

- Do this at the same time each day.

- Test for five consecutive days.

The basal temperature should be between 97.8 and 98.2°F and 36.6 and 36.8°C. If the Test shows the temperature to be consistently below these levels then the Patient's Doctor should be advised. (Note: drinking alcohol also lowers the reading).

Note: Men may undertake this test on any sequence of days. For women who are menstruating the temperature is best measured on days two, three, four, five, and six of their period. Before puberty and after menopause any five days will do. (See Table 8 The Barnes Axillary Temperature Test)

Remember that any system that is over-worked or over-stimulated will eventually under-function or close down.

Hormonal Disorders: Suggestions for Discussion with Patient as Part of Developing the Treatment Plan

- Explore ways in which the Patient is able to reduce stress and undertake gentle exercise. Also have enough sleep; and avoid all stimulants.

- 'Anti-thyroid antibodies' are often due to a gluten allergy, therefore if the Patient has an underactive thyroid it is worth testing for food allergies. (Holford P, 2005)

- Consider the diet (as for constipation), and need to avoid sugar and refined carbohydrates.

- Essential fatty acids are important, therefore suggest oily fish, two or three times weekly, plenty of seeds, walnuts, almonds, and brazil nuts. The oils or supplements of evening primrose or borage oil (omega-6) or linseed oil (omega-3).

- Consider digestive disturbance and digestive enzymes. Drink plenty of distilled water.

- Recommend liver detoxification.

- Consider extra calcium, B12, B3 (niacin) and C. Discuss supplements designed for adrenal exhaustion or, as appropriate, thyroid imbalance.

- Be mindful of hypoglycaemia, consider testing blood-sugar levels.

Hypoglycaemia is a deficiency of glucose in the blood stream, which causes muscular weakness and fatigue, mental confusion, and sweating. If severe it may lead to hypoglycaemic coma. When too

131

much glucose is present in the body the pancreas increases the amount of insulin being produced.

The Glucose Tolerance Test (GTT) is the standard medical blood test for hypoglycaemia and is performed in the morning following an evening of fasting. The blood test is to determine the 'fasting' blood-sugar level. After this, the Patient is given a glucose solution to drink and after an hour another blood sample is taken. Five more blood samples are taken at hourly intervals. In hypoglycaemic Patients the natural rise will be followed by a rapid drop below the normal fasting range. The faster that it drops, and the degree to which it drops, determines the severity of the condition. High levels of blood glucose (hyperglycaemia) are very toxic.

The glycaemic index (GI), is a practical way of evaluating and measuring the carbohydrates we may consume and their respective glucose levels. The greater the blood-sugar level the greater the insulin response. (See Table 1, Diet and Nutrition Section).

Hypoglycaemia: Suggestions for Discussion with the Patient as Part of Developing the Treatment Plan.

- Exploration of lifestyle, dietary habits, dietary abuses, and degree of stress. High GI-index carbohydrates must be avoided. Hypoglycaemic Patients may also be suffering with Candidiasis.

- The need to exclude, absolutely, sugar of any kind; or glucose, treacle, chocolate, sweets, cake, or biscuits. (As a concession, a maximum of half a teaspoon of honey daily).

- Refined grains are valueless, that is: avoid white flower, white rice, processed breakfast cereal, pies, pastries, and avoid breads. Only genuine whole rye or stone-ground loaves are suitable. In fact, the Patient would benefit from avoiding yeast until feeling stronger. Suggest rice cakes.

- Discuss need to avoid: fruit juice drinks and coffee. The consumption of alcohol and salt must be seriously restricted, and consumption of fresh fruit juices should be limited. Two fresh vegetable juices of half water half juice will be a useful cleansing addition to the diet.

- Include a low-GI carbohydrate at every meal.

- High fibre and protein-rich foods and six small meals per day making certain that a substantial breakfast is part of the plan (dried fruits like sultanas can be added to breakfast), and ensure provision of good-quality snacks (nuts, seeds, and a very small amount of dried fruits only). Suggest brown rice snacks, thin slices of rye bread, carrot and celery sticks, a little cheese, and good quality probiotic yoghurt.

- Supplements to be considered will include chromium, which is required for metabolism of sugar. Zinc is a constituent of insulin and is important in both hypo/hyperglycaemic conditions. Good sources include: whole grains, seeds, nuts. Chelated zinc is indicated as a supplement. Note that magnesium deficiencies can lead to rapid drops in blood-sugar and most hypoglycaemics are deficient in this mineral.

- Stress to be reduced. Consider long walks, and massage.

INDICATIONS GROUP FOUR

Digestive Disorders:

Gastritis is an inflammation or irritation of the lining of the stomach. It is not a single disease. Gastritis is a condition that has many causes but common to all sufferers of gastritis is pain or discomfort in the upper part of the abdomen, which is sometimes called dyspepsia. It can be a brief condition or long lasting. Up to 10% of people who go to a hospital emergency department with abdominal pain have gastritis. Pain occurs in the left upper portion of the abdomen and in the back and is described as 'going straight through you', from belly to back. Patients also use the terms burning, gnawing, aching, sore, sharp, or cutting to describe their pain. Other symptoms include: belching, nausea, vomiting, bloating, feeling of fullness, and heartburn.

Often there is constipation, and occasionally there may be diarrhoea due to intestinal catarrh. In more severe cases, bleeding may occur in the stomach, severe stomach pain, vomiting blood, and bloody bowel movements or dark, sticky, very foul-smelling bowel movements. Any or all of these symptoms can occur suddenly, particularly in older people. A frequent cause is dietary indiscretion: overeating, eating rich foods, processed foods, excessive consumption of strong tea/coffee, alcoholic drinks, and poorly combined foods. The majority of people recover. Depending upon the factors that affect the Patient's stomach lining, symptoms may flare-up from time to time.

Gastritis: Suggestions for Discussion with the Patient as Part of Developing the Treatment Plan.

- The mainstay of prevention is to avoid the things that irritate or inflame. Gastric ulcers are caused by the action of acid, pepsin, and bile on the stomach mucosa.

- Avoid alcohol, gluten, citrus, monosodium-glutamate, milk and dairy products, caffeine sources, deep-fried foods, margarine. Use extra-virgin olive oil as main fat and increase intake of omega-3 fatty acids.

- As with the majority of diseases, lifestyle, anxiety, prolonged tension, and stress are often part of the symptom picture.

- Supported by colon hydrotherapy, part of the treatment plan may include: fasting for a couple of days with warm water drinks in order to allow the toxic conditions causing the inflammation to subside.

- Thereafter, gradually embark upon a balanced diet consisting of fresh fruit, vegetables, and grain.

- Include in the treatment plan the suggestions discussed regarding IBS, especially digestive enzymes (take before meals), chlorophyll supplement, and avoid irritants.

- If heartburn or indigestion is present, this can be eased by drinking lemon juice and/or cider vinegar or use a charcoal supplement.

Food Allergies and allergies in general are disorders in which the body becomes hypersensitive to particular antigens, called allergens. These provoke a characteristic symptom whenever they are inhaled, ingested, injected, or otherwise contacted. The word 'allergy' means there is an allergic reaction when body tissues are sensitive to given allergens. A patient may also experience an intolerance or sensitivity to a substance that may not provoke an obvious symptom, but could be associated with a chronic condition

Almost any part of the body can be affected by allergies, although it is primarily the skin, mucous membranes, lungs, and gastrointestinal tract that are affected. Reactions can be caused by a wide range of substances, sources, or conditions. These include (there are literally thousands of possibilities): pollens from trees and grasses, mould spores, dust, cosmetics, sprays, animal hair, plants, tobacco, serums, vaccines, heat, cold, environmental chemicals, food additives, and, of course, many different foods.

Foods that commonly cause allergic reactions or intolerances are cow's milk, citrus fruit, wheat, sea-foods, chocolate, strawberries, yeast, E numbers, and eggs. Symptoms include: recurring headaches, depression, neuralgia, conjunctivitis, eczema, hay fever, diarrhoea, urticaria (hives, itchy rash, weals), vomiting, constipation, asthma, swelling of face and eyes. Seen from a naturopathic perspective, allergic symptoms represent the body endeavouring to detoxify an overly congested system/s. (See Table 8a, Food Additives: Function and Effects. Main B, 2007).

Note: 'when the diet is clean, the stress level is low, and the eliminative functions are working well, we will exhibit minimal, if any symptoms'. (Haas E, 2006).

Food Allergies/Sensitivity: Suggestions for Discussion with the Patient as Part of Discussing the Treatment Plan.

- Colon hydrotherapy and detoxification diets are recommended, including a food allergy test. (See Useful Addresses).

- Eliminate cow's milk and milk products and substitute other calcium sources.

- Eliminate other foods accordingly following allergy test.

- Decrease protein toward 10% of daily calorific intake and replace animal protein as much as possible with plant protein. (Weil A, 2001).

- If the Patient is not allergic to citrus fruit then half of a fresh lime squeezed into a glass of lukewarm water to be taken daily may be recommended. Take first thing in the morning for several months. This remedy helps flush the system of toxins and is said to also act as an anti-allergic agent.

- Alternatively five drops of castor oil in half a cup of vegetable juice, first thing in the morning, has been found to be beneficial for allergies of the intestinal tract, skin, and nasal passages. (See Indications Concerning Skin Disorders).

INDICATIONS GROUP FIVE

Parasite Infections:

Parasite Infection. No matter how long the symptom list of a Patient may have, it is likely that many are signs that parasite infection is present. Such symptoms include: chronic fatigue, insomnia, sexual dysfunction in men, bloating, the loss of appetite, fast heartbeat, itchy anus, eyes, nose, and ears. Symptoms also include eating more than normal but still feeling hungry, lethargy, problems with menstrual cycle, diarrhoea, anaemia, cancer, allergies.

A parasite is a living thing that lives in, or on, another living organism. Some will interfere with bodily functions; others destroy host tissues and release toxins into the body thus affecting health and causing serious acute and chronic disease.

Acute parasitic infection is characterized by abdominal distress, diarrhoea, burning sensations, and fluid loss. With chronic conditions there may be alternating periods of constipation and diarrhoea, abdominal distension, and intestinal cramping, and the sudden urge to eliminate. There will be malabsorption of nutrients, IBS symptoms, blood-sugar fluctuations, emaciation, or overweight.

Moreover **parasites are not always intestinal worms.** Parasites can be in any part of the body, for example, in the head, blood, thyroid glands, mucous in the chest, other bodily systems, and organs, but especially the bowel. Parasite infection is highly contagious and casual contact can lead to infection. Infection comes from various sources, for example, contaminated water, improperly washed or undercooked food, transmission from pets, poor sanitation, soil, vegetables, fruit, and packaged food.

Human parasites include also fungi such as yeasts and moulds. The most common is ***candida albicans.*** (We all have yeast in our digestive tract but when it grows out of control it is called candidiasis.

Parasites include:

Bacteria, a group of organisms that are more primitive than animal and plant cells, include *shigella* bacteria, which can cause dreadful constipation, and the *salmonella* bacteria responsible for food poisoning, gastroenteritis, and septicaemia. There are some 4,000 different bacteria in the healthy human intestine.

Viruses are parasites which are capable of replication but only in living cells. The Epstein-Barre virus (causing sore throat, swollen lymph glands, and temperature), belonging to the herpes virus, is believed to come from the pancreatic fluke worm. (After primary infection all the herpes viruses enter a state of latency).

Protozoa are single-celled parasites, for example, *Plasmodium,* which causes malaria.

Worms are any member of several groups of soft-bodied legless animals, including: **flatworms** (tapeworms and flukes) and **roundworms** (threadworms, pinworms, and hookworms).

Roundworms like the *filaria* worm penetrate the intestinal wall and cause diarrhoea and nausea, and migrate through the body. The most common roundworm is the *ascaris* worm (commonly found in cats and dogs) and causes colicky pain and urticaria. When in the intestines the *ascaris* worm deposits 20,000 eggs per day, they hatch, and then penetrate the liver, they move to the heart and then lungs, eggs are coughed up and swallowed thus entering the gastrointestinal tract until a sexually mature worm emerges, and the first eggs appear in the stool. Whilst in the abdominal phase abdominal pain, vomiting, and enteritis can occur. The round worm *enterobius vermicularis* crawls out of the anus at night and causes itching and inevitable scratching!!

The **flatworm** *ancylostoma* hooks itself into the jejunum and sucks the blood necessary for its metabolism and respiration. There is an association between hook worms and ulcerative colitis and unclarified occult blood found in the faeces. (Occult blood is blood present in such small quantities that it can only be detected microscopically or by chemical testing).

With tapeworms their eggs are eaten, say on a poorly washed salad, the larvae hatch and then burrow into their favourite organ where the body encases it with a cyst. They come out of their cyst and attach themselves to the intestine and start laying their eggs. The *fasciolopsis buskii,* the fluke flatworm, causes chronic infections, inflammation, ulceration, haemorrhage, and abscesses.

Moulds produce some of the most toxic substances known, called mycotoxins. A tiny amount can incapacitate a part of the liver. Aflotoxin (a specific toxin caused by the mould *aspergillus flavus*) can cause a type of hepatitis or even liver cancer. It is associated with the common peanut, may contaminate other nuts, as well as corn, wheat, and barley.

Parasite Infection: Suggestions for Discussion with the

Patient as Part of Developing the Treatment Plan

- Consider a recommended treatment strategy combining colon hydrotherapy, liver and kidney cleanse, general detoxification, and a parasite-removal treatment.

- The use of herbs and foods to facilitate healing and use pure products, keep meals simple, combining fresh organic foods, avoiding sugars and avoiding processed foods. (See discussion regarding the treatment for *candida albicans*).

- Avoiding situations that could lead to parasite infection by following precautions suggested: drink clean filtered water. Chlorination does not kill all parasites. It is advisable to boil drinking water.

- Always wash fresh produce carefully and thoroughly, especially fruit and vegetables.

- Always wash hands thoroughly after the toilet and ALWAYS before preparing a meal.

- If the Patient eats meat, then the requirement to ensure it is cooked thoroughly.

- The limiting or cutting out of synthetic/artificially flavoured food and packaged food.

- Discuss the benefits of building and toning of the intestines with colon hydrotherapy, garlic, herbs, fibre, exercise, rest, fasting and cleansing diets.

- Start taking *probiotics*, these are concentrated sources of beneficial bacteria. The best probiotics contain *lactobacillus acidophilus* and *bifidobacteria*, which are normally resident in the gut. Note: the healthy bowel has around 85% friendly lactobacillus, and 15% unfriendly gas-producing *bacillus coli.*

- Ways of developing and maintaining a healthy lifestyle in order to guard against parasites.

(See section on 'Cleansing and Detoxification Diets, Including Fasting, Parasite Cleanse, Kidney and Liver Cleanse).

Candida albicans is a yeast, and *candidiasis* is an overgrowth of that yeast. *Candida albicans* is quite normal in a healthy person. When an imbalance in intestinal flora occurs, *candidiasis* can become pathogenic, grow out of control, and crowd out beneficial flora which perform an essential part in a wide range of the body's needs, including the detoxification of harmful chemicals. These toxins then damage body tissues and cause many of the symptoms familiar to *candidiasis* sufferers.

The range of symptoms is large and includes: unexplained fatigue, abdominal bloating, food cravings, particularly for sugar and bread, food and chemical sensitivities, rectal itching, fungal infections of the skin or nails, athlete's foot, psoriasis, acne, recurrent thrush, or cystitis.

Causes of *candida albicans* overgrowth include: antibiotic use, birth control pill, hormone replacement therapy, steroids, immune-suppressive drugs and weakened immunity, diet high in refined carbohydrates and sugar, prolonged stress, insufficiency of hydrochloric acid in the stomach, pancreatic enzyme deficiency. (Jacobs G, 1997).

Once established, **candidiasis alters the pH balance** of the intestines. This then creates the wrong acidity for beneficial bacteria to maintain their colonies. Symptoms usually start in the digestive tract or the vagina. **Vaginal thrush** is an overgrowth of yeast that can lead to extremely uncomfortable and unpleasant symptoms around the vagina such as: itching, soreness, pain, swelling of the vagina and vulva, often with a yeast-smelling discharge.

Candida albicans: Suggestions for Discussion with the Patient as Part of Developing the Treatment Plan

- That detoxification be recommended at the start of a treatment plan. This is supported by a *candidiasis* control diet, probiotics, and natural anti-fungal food, for example, fresh raw organic garlic chopped and washed down with water before a meal and plenty of pumpkin seeds. Or, Candicidin, which is a non-chemical antifungal that includes: oregano, cloves, ginger, grapefruit seed oil.

- A programme of colon hydrotherapy treatments being an essential part of the treatment plan.

Cystitis is inflammation of the bladder. **There are two types**. The most common form is **bacterial cystitis,** caused by the *escherichia coli* bacteria, which normally lives in and around the anus, entering the urethra. Males and females are affected, although it is most common in women. Symptoms include: burning and stinging pain when urinating, frequent need to pass small amounts of urine; feeling an urgency to pass urine when the bladder is empty; and passing cloudy/dark urine that may have a strong smell.

The second type of cystitis is **interstitial cystitis,** which involves inflammation of the bladder but without bacteria being present. The cause is uncertain but could be a type of allergy or deficiency in the bladder lining. The sexually transmitted disease of *Chlamydia* can cause symptoms similar to cystitis.

Cystitis: Suggestions for Discussion with the Patient as Part of Developing the Treatment Plan.

- Colon hydrotherapy, detoxification, kidney cleanse, as part of the treatment plan.
- Avoid all forms of sugar, and all caffeine sources.
- Also drinking plenty of water and/or cranberry juice, (ensure no citric acid present in the cranberry juice or could inflame the condition).
- The need to empty the bladder according to urges to go; avoiding caffeine, sexual intercourse, spicy food.

Halitosis (bad-smelling breath) is often caused by periodontal disease (in the tissues surrounding the teeth), constipation, indigestion, and infective conditions of the lungs. Most halitosis stems from bacterial production of odiferous compounds.

Halitosis: Suggestions for Discussion with the Patient as Part of the Development of the Treatment Plan

- Approach as per suggestions for the treatment of parasites and *candida albicans.*

- General measures to treat may include zinc, as this will reduce the concentration of volatile sulphur compounds in the mouth, and measures to deal with the underlying cause. Tea Tree, cloves, peppermint all have antibacterial properties and are therefore worthy of consideration in the treatment plan.

INDICATIONS GROUP SIX

Skin Disorders:

Skin problems range between severe disorders such as eczema and psoriasis and less severe disorders like dry skin and dandruff, and there can be many factors involved. Naturopathy and natural therapeutics are often called upon to treat skin problems and these can be among the most difficult to treat. The skin is the largest eliminatory organ and is sometimes called the 'third kidney'. The skin is therefore often an indicator that the normal organs of elimination and detoxification are not coping. Many skin problems are also linked to parasite infection but as we know from our studies so far there is rarely one single cause of any health problem.

Eczema is almost certainly one of the commonest skin disorders. It can appear anywhere on the body with symptoms such as: itching, redness, inflammation, soreness, weeping and scaling skin. It can run in families, and may accompany other conditions like asthma and hay fever. There is potential for confusion when discussing eczema as there are different types with different causes. For example, **atopic eczema** is seen as a genetic condition. However, a person with atopic eczema is more likely to develop allergies.

Discoid eczema is often caused by dry skin becoming infected with the *staphylococcus aureus* bacteria. The bacteria secrete toxins that make the eczema worse and cracks in the skin can develop into deeper fissures. Therefore, the eradication of the bacteria is necessary if the treatment plan is to be successful.

142

Allergic contact dermatitis is eczema caused by an allergy. When the body has developed an allergy to a chemical, or irritant that comes into contact with the skin the immune system will react to it. An allergy can arise from almost anything!

Varicose eczema is eczema found on the lower legs above the ankle. The role that varicose veins have in varicose eczema is unclear.

Eczema: Suggestions for Discussion with the Patient as Part of Developing the Treatment Plan

- The importance in treating various eczemas for the Patient to be mindful of known and possible 'triggers' or irritants, and eradicate them, as far is possible, from diet and environment. Examples include: dairy products, soaps, perfumes, and many household chemicals. Include issues discussed under 'Allergies'.

- Increase omega-3 fatty acids, and discuss a diet low in saturated fat, but with sufficient essential fats from seeds and their cold- pressed oils.

- The lack of linolenic acid (an essential fatty acid) can result in eczema. Linolenic acid is found in most plant oils, for example: canola, safflower, sesame, and sunflower. All are best used on salads and cooked grains. (Is also found in wheatgerm and oat germ).

- Eczema can be eased by taking one to three dessert spoonfuls of quality cold-pressed vegetable oil per day).

- As with all conditions, detoxification and colon hydrotherapy will help support the body in its fight against and allergens and pathogens of all kinds.

Psoriasis, often runs in families and commonly occurs in adolescence. The disease may be very severe, affecting much of the skin. While psychological stress usually exacerbates the condition a noted event that sometimes precipitates the disease is a preceding *streptococcal* bacteria infection. If the liver is overwhelmed by an increasing number of toxins, including from *candida albicans* and other bowel toxicity, psoriasis may become much worse.

It is suggested that discussions regarding the **treatment plan** explore colon hydrotherapy and liver detoxification as being important parts of the treatment plan. Plus antioxidant vitamins A, C, and E and zinc, which are crucial to healthy skin and as such are particularly helpful along with fatty acids mentioned above. Also taking cod liver oil or evening primrose oil has been found to be helpful.

Acne is inflammation of the subaceous glands that not only produce sebum (which helps keep the skin supple), but also has antibacterial properties. Acne is estimated to torment 80% of adolescents, causing hurt, embarrassment, emotional pain and low self-esteem likely to affect school and college performance and no doubt job opportunities. Toxicity, from parasites is often the root cause, and foods can aggravate, for example dairy products and sugar. The bacteria involved with acne are called *Propionibacterium acnes* that colonise the sebum in the sebaceous glands and ducts. Discussions regarding the **treatment plan** to explore:

- Colon hydrotherapy, parasite cleanse and kidney and liver cleanse will kill the parasites, remove the toxins, and will certainly be found to be restorative. Refer to other suggestions within this group of symptoms, especially supplements containing vitamin A, C, and zinc, with vitamin E for wound healing.

Be not too alarmed, even a meticulously clean life will be exposed to bacteria, some are harmful, some are neutral, and some are essential to a healthy life. It is only when an imbalance occurs that problems occur!

'The bacteria found associated with acute, sub-acute and chronic diseases are not the primary causes and instigators of these abnormal processes but rather the product of pathogenic conditions and agents and instigators of these abnormal processes'. (Lindlahr H, I996).

INDICATIONS GROUP SEVEN

Other Chronic Conditions:

Remember: the term 'chronic' is describing a disease or symptom/s of long-term duration and persistence, but does not imply anything about the severity of a disease or symptoms.

Chronic Fatigue Syndrome (CFS) and Myalgic Encephalo-myelitis (ME). Myalgic means aches and pains, encephalomyelitis means inflammation of the brain and spinal cord and are viewed by some experts as two separate conditions. Others say they are the same but that symptoms can vary. CFS/ME is a complex illness characterized by severe, prolonged fatigue in addition to numerous other symptoms including: pharyngitis, fever, pain in the muscles and joints, headaches, sleep disorders, difficulty in concentration, and short-term memory loss. Is twice as common in women and usually presents between the early-twenties and mid-forties.

Diagnosis is made on the basis of symptoms, although blood tests may be undertaken to rule out anaemia, underactive thyroid, liver, and kidney problems. All tests will show normal in people with CFS/ME with symptoms being present for six months.

As there is only limited success with conventional treatments it is understandable that Patients may use complementary medicine Practitioners. In most cases, symptoms take a fluctuating course and the long-term outlook is variable. The severity of symptoms will also range from mild, moderate, severe to very severe. Depression is quite common and can make symptoms worse.

Cause is uncertain although there is a widely held view that chronic infection with viruses such as Epstein-Barre virus (sore throat, swollen lymph-glands, temperature), human herpes virus 6, and cylomegalovirus contribute to the development of CFS/ME.

(Research suggests viruses are dormant within the body and become active when the immune system becomes compromised. Stress and emotional difficulties are also believed to be contributing factors.

Progressing with colon hydrotherapy as part of the **treatment plan will depend upon the given severity of the condition.** Stress reduction, muscle relaxation, general relaxation, yoga, and exercise (as appropriate) may be considered as part of the treatment plan. The co-enzyme Q10, which is a compound found naturally in the mitochondria, the energy-producing centre of our cells, has been found to be helpful. (Q10 is also an antioxidant). Discuss nutrients high in vitamin C and B complex, iron and magnesium, multimineral and multivitamin supplements, and to follow recommendations for an optimum health diet. Consider hormonal disorder options.

Asthma is a chronic condition involving the respiratory system in which the bronchial airways narrow, changing in severity over short periods of time, which leads to coughing, wheezing, and difficulty in breathing. Asthma may, for example, be precipitated by exposure to allergens (typically: dairy products, house-dust mites, household pets, household chemicals, food additives, medications, exertion, infections, pollen, mould spores, and emotions).

Asthma is often triggered in response to more than one or more factors. An acute exacerbation of asthma is called an 'asthma attack' caused by a complex interaction of genetic and environmental factors.

As with allergy, the most effective part of the **treatment plan** is for the Patient to be clear about triggers and limiting or removing exposure to them. **Follow recommendations under 'Allergies'.** Attention in the press (and clinic) has been drawn to the increasing prevalence of asthma, especially in children. Similar to others who suffer from chronic diseases asthmatics often use complementary treatments. For example, the Buteyko method, a therapy based upon breathing exercises, showed, in the trial group, a reduction in the use of medication and inhaled steroid use after six months.

(McHugh P et al, 2003). Hatha yoga practice has for centuries taught a complete range of breathing patterns to advance energy, create balance of energies, relax the body, and improve health. Colon hydrotherapy and the cleansing the body of toxins will only help matters.

Arthritis (which means inflammation of the joints) occurs in various forms, the most frequent being osteoarthritis, a degenerative disease, usually occurring in older age, causing pain, and stiffness in the joints. The skilled colon hydrotherapist may be limited in what is possible with musculo-skeletal difficulties of Patients but may have much to offer in giving gentle relief to bowel problems. They may also provide suggestions regarding the Patient's nutritional wellbeing. Recent Government reports showed that nutritional deficiencies in older people had become a major concern for the health and social care service professions. (Department of Health Reports, 1998 and 2007).

Rheumatoid arthritis is an autoimmune disease. Of the diseases and conditions discussed so far in this book, **autoimmune diseases include: coeliac disease, Crohn's disease, and rheumatoid arthritis. Diseases suspected or theorised to be autoimmune also include interstitial cystitis, psoriasis, and ulcerative colitis.** Rheumatoid arthritis is a disease that affects not only the joints but also the muscles, tendons, and other tissues of the body. Symptoms include, pain, swelling in the joints, and stiffness and food intolerances can aggravate the condition.

Autoimmune disorders are diagnosed, evaluated, and monitored through a combination of autoantibody blood tests, blood tests to measure inflammation and organ function, clinical presentation, and through non-laboratory examinations like X-rays. There is currently no cure. Many people experience flare-ups and temporary remissions in symptoms. Others experience chronic symptoms, or a progressive worsening. **The treatment goals are to relieve symptoms, minimise organ and tissue damage, and preserve organ function.**

The Treatment Plan discussions to explore: anti-inflammatory approaches and the range of detoxification options including colon hydrotherapy. It is essential that Patient's consider the benefits of an **alkaline-forming diet** in order to produce the required level of alkalinity in the blood, and therefore less acid. In severe cases it may be advisable for the Patient to consider adopting a raw vegetable juice therapy three times a day for about a week. Calcium, taken in the form of calcium lactate, can also relieve joint pain. Ginger and turmeric are useful for their anti-inflammatory effects.

Gout, although not an autoimmune disease, involves painful attacks of arthritis and often the first joint to be affected (in 70% of cases) is the big toe. Excess uric acid in the blood and tissues, with crystals of urate forming around the joints and kidneys (the end products of protein metabolism) are indicative of gout and affects five times as many men as women.(www.ukgoutsociety.org).

Patient's who are overweight, eat diets rich in protein, and drink large quantities of alcohol have an increased risk of developing the disease, and therefore must reduce the level of alcohol intake, eat less red meat, kidneys, liver, and seafood. (Diuretics can also interfere with normal excretion of uric acid).

Treatment Plan discussions will be similar to those for Arthritis and to include, as appropriate, colon hydrotherapy. RECOMMEND MOVING TOWARDS A HIGH ALKALINE DIET.

INDICATIONS GROUP EIGHT

Other Relevant Conditions:

Headaches and Migraines. Most of us suffer at one time or another, and some people are especially susceptible. There are several different types of headache and these can sometimes be a symptom of a serious disease so if accompanied by, for example, fever, rash, seizure numbness, or speaking problems, seek medical help immediately.

Tension headaches are the most common causing a dull throbbing pain and a feeling of pressure or tightness in the scalp or neck.

Migraine is another relatively common form of headache, although around 60% of people who regularly complain of headaches have migraine. (Channel 4, Complementary Medicine, Headaches and Migraine, 2007). Symptoms include severe throbbing pain usually concentrated on one side of the head, nausea or vomiting, dislike of noise or bright light, and may be preceded by visual disturbances, stiff neck, and yawning.

Cluster headaches are another type, so-called because they occur in bouts, often around the same time of day. They cause a piercing pain in and around the eye, which may be watery and inflamed.

The exact causes of headaches or migraine are not fully understood. However, muscular tension, stress and tension, food intolerance, hormonal changes, changes in the weather, lack of food, lack of sleep, and alcohol use, are among the triggers. **Treatment Plan** to involve: colon hydrotherapy, detoxification, food-allergy/intollerance testing, and massage and relaxation are likely to be further aspects for consideration as part of the treatment programme. Monitor possible triggers.

Sleep Disorders often accompany many of the diseases and conditions discussed above and are increasingly being seen as a problem in our high stress and fast-paced life styles. We often go to bed with our mind racing, busy with thoughts, and we find it difficult to sleep. Sleep disorders include: difficulty in falling to sleep; often waking up during the night; waking up too early in the morning; unrefreshing sleep, choking, gasping (apnoea), and snoring.

In establishing the **Treatment Plan** the hydrotherapist may involve the Patient in 'self-diagnosis' by asking them to pay attention to their living habits, life style, and daily routines as an important way of identifying possible causes. For example, eating late, consuming stimulants like coffee or alcohol, mood swings, medicines, uncomfortable bed, and poorly ventilated bedroom. Also explore ways which aim to: improve bedtimes and regularise sleeping hours, relieve stress, and incorporate bedtime rituals, with opportunities to relax and sip a herbal tea as cues to the body that it is now time to slow down.

Back Pain is second only to the common cold for time off work. Back pain is a symptom. Pain arising from other organs may be felt in the back and is called referred pain and may for example, come from intra-abdominal disorders such as kidney disease, an over-burdened liver, or muscular and skeletal problems. **The Treatment Plan may consider:** hot and cold fomentations, applied for four and one minute respectively. Such has been found to be of value in long-standing conditions such as back pain, and will stimulate circulatory and lymphatic drainage in numerous other conditions. Include colon hydrotherapy, detoxification method, and liaise as appropriate with other relevant professionals, for example, chiropractor.

Comment

Colon Hydrotherapy and other complementary and naturopathic approaches may not always provide a greater likelihood of 'cure' than more conventional interventions. However, they can certainly support the Patient in understanding particular symptoms and causes and enable them to understand and facilitate their body's own adaptive and regulatory processes; thus, enabling them to cope more effectively with their particular condition, and avoid unnecessary despair and anxiety through the support and guidance given to them by their Practitioner. Remember also the benefits of meaningful relationships, activity, self-esteem, and the incomparable benefits of being outside, in the air, and in the sunshine. AS A PRIORITY, REDUCE ACID-FORMING FOODS, feelings and behaviours will also alter, for the better!

Furthermore, through given treatment plans Practitioners have the opportunity to encourage preventive treatments, as the well-known adage suggests: 'prevention is better than cure'!

The Five Systems of Elimination

The most important elimination systems are the **colon** (a term which is used inter-changeably with the bowel and large intestine), **urinary system, lungs, and skin.** The **lymph system** works with these four systems by serving as 'rubbish collector' by carrying the metabolic by-products and other accumulated cellular waste from the tissues to the four elimination organs mentioned. In the healthy adult these systems eliminate around a kilo of waste material daily.

We know that if any one of these systems is under-functioning an accumulation of toxic wastes in the body will result, and toxins will be forced into the bloodstream to settle in those organs and tissues that have the least resistance to toxic materials.

It is a Course Entry Requirement that students have passed an examination in anatomy and physiology. The discussion that follows provides information on the five systems in order to provide the Practitioner with a useful reference and revision medium to inform direct practice.

Colon cleansing, and kidney regimens and liver regimens cleansing routines, are important concerning overall body cleansing and detoxification, which we discuss later. First, let us consider the five systems in order to demonstrate their relatedness to colon hydrotherapy treatment.

The Colon

For colon hydrotherapists it is axiomatic that the part of human anatomy and physiology they must have a comprehensive knowledge of is the bowel. So, let us revisit this subject. (See Figure 1)

The large intestine is mainly responsible for:

- Storing waste.

- Reclaiming water, maintaining the water balance, and solidifying the faeces.

- Absorbing some vitamins, such as vitamin K (necessary for normal blood clotting). At this point some electrolytes, like sodium, magnesium, and chloride are left as indigestible carbohydrates known as dietary fibre.

- Absorbing toxic substances to be sent to the liver to be detoxified.

- Breaking down undigested carbohydrates, proteins, and amino acids into products that can be expelled by the faeces or absorbed and detoxified by the liver.

- The mucosa secretes mucous that lubricates the colon and also protects the mucosa.

- Provides muscular contractions, (haustral churning, peristalsis, mass peristalsis and defecation), which moves the contents of the colon from haustrum to haustrum, and also provides contractions of circular and longitudinal muscles to move contents along the length of the colon into the sigmoid colon and rectum by strong peristaltic waves so the faeces can be eliminated by contractions of the sigmoid colon and rectum.

- Provides for bacterial activity, known as gut flora, as part of the breakdown of chyme and elimination processes, releasing hydrogen, carbon dioxide, and methane gas. These gases contribute to flatus (gas) in the colon. The bacteria break down some of the fibre for their own nourishment and create acetate, propionate, and butyrate (products in the bioconversion of organic matter to methane and carbon dioxide) as waste products, which in turn are used by the cell lining of the colon for nourishment. The breakdown of amino acids into simpler substances creates indole and skatole (formed in the rumen region of the stomach from the degradation of dietary protein), which contributes to the odour of stools. Bacteria also decompose bilirubin, (which gives faeces their brown colour) and is a product of the blood pigment haem, which contains iron and is linked to the protein globin. Haemoglobin, remember, is the medium by which oxygen is transported within the body.

The large intestine is 1.5m (5 feet), and has the following parts: the **caecum and vermiform appendix, the ascending colon, the transverse colon, the descending colon, the pelvic or sigmoid colon, and the rectum.**

The large intestine is part of the alimentary tract and starts at the entrance of the terminal part of the ileum into the caecum and ends at the anus, which is the opening of the rectum to the exterior.

The **caecum** is a dilated sac situated in the right iliac fossa into which the ileum enters at the **ileocaecal valve**. The mucous membrane is so arranged at this point, together with the sphincter muscle, it acts as a valve that permits the contents of the ileum, chyme, to enter the caecum but preventing their return into the ileum. The caecum has the largest diameter of the large intestine, 7.62cm (3 inches), and is the least motile. The worm-like tube attached to the blind end of the caecum, is the **vermiform appendix.** It is around 8.89cm long (3.5 inches), and lies, in the right iliac fossa. It is lined by mucous membrane and contains lymphoid tissue in its walls, and produces a germicide-type secretion into the caecum. Inflammation of this structure is referred to as appendicitis.

The **ascending colon,** approximately 20 to 25cm (8 inches) long, passes upward through the right lumbar region and is held in position on the posterior abdominal wall by peritoneum. It reaches the undersurface of the liver, where it turns sharply to the left at the right or **hepatic flexure** and becomes the **transverse colon,** 45cm in length, (16 to 20 inches). **This region exhibits the most colonic movement.** It extends across the abdominal cavity as a loop that may fall well below the umbilicus.

The **transverse colon** lies in the fold of peritoneum that extends downwards from the greater curvature of the stomach called the great omentum. It is, therefore, freely moveable within the abdominal cavity. It reaches its left extremity and comes in contact with the spleen, where it turns sharply downwards at the left or **splenic flexure** to continue as the **descending colon**, approximately 10 to 15cm.

The colon turns to the midline at the iliac crest in a form resembling the letter S. The descending colon passes downwards in the left lumbar region. It is anchored to the posterior abdominal wall by the peritoneum and, therefore, like the ascending colon is not moveable. The descending colon is approximately 27cm in length (10 to 12 inches). The area of the descending colon from the **sigmoid flexure** is the **sigmoid colon**, approximately 40cm in length, (16 inches).

The sigmoid colon is the continuation of the descending colon and, having a mesentery (a double layer of peritoneum) is moveable. It lies mainly in the pelvic cavity and passes into the **rectum**, approximately 20cm in length, (7 to 8 inches). Three semilunar valves, the **Valves of Houston**, are present in the mucosal layer of the rectum, which slows faecal movement through this region. The rectum is not designed to be a reservoir, but is normally empty unless defecation is occurring. Therefore, stool does not enter the rectum from the colon on a continuous basis, but as a result of mass motility movements. Usually, the descending colon and sigmoid colon evacuate at the same time.

The final part of the rectum, approximately 7cm (2 to 3 inches) long is referred to as the **anal canal** and opens to the exterior of the **anus** through which faecal material is voided. This opening is guarded by a sphincter muscle, the anal sphincter. An external sphincter muscle is located at the distal (nearest the exterior) end of the canal and an internal sphincter at its proximal end. The former is under the control of the will so that it can be relaxed when it is desired to empty the contents of the rectum.

The lining of the anal canal is not mucous (a surface of moist membrane) but of squamous epithelium (flat or scale-like membrane). Several blood vessels are present in this region and their inflammation is known as piles or **haemorrhoids.**

The colon, like the small intestine has four 'coats': peritoneal or serous (containing a fluid resembling serum), muscular, submucous, and mucous. The characteristic feature, however, is that the longitudinal muscles do not form a continuous layer over the whole gut but are arranged in three separate bands. These bands are somewhat shorter than the length of the large intestine, which accounts for its sacculated appearance. When the longitudinal fibres reach the rectum they spread out over its whole surface. The mucous membrane contains no villi and is not thrown into folds like the small intestine. It is lined with columnar epithelium, which function primarily to absorb water. Solitary lymphatic nodules are found in the mucosa.

The portal circulation (circulation inside the abdominal cavity) concerns the blood that is supplied and removed from the organs of digestion and its conveyance to the liver.

Blood comes from the following branches of the abdominal aorta:

- The coeliac axis artery supplying the stomach, spleen, the pancreas, and the liver.

- The superior mesenteric artery to the small intestine and the first part of the large intestine (ascending colon).

- The inferior mesenteric artery to the rest of the large intestine and the rectum.

- Two-thirds of the transverse colon is perfused (the passage of fluid through tissue) by the middle colic artery (branch of the superior mesenteric artery). The final third is supplied by branches of the inferior mesenteric artery. For the descending colon, arterial supply comes via the left colic artery, sigmoid, and superior haemorrhoidal artery.

These arteries all break up into capillaries in the actual organs which they supply and these unite to form veins.

Venous drainage usually mirrors colonic arterial supply, with the inferior mesenteric vein draining into the splenic vein, and the superior mesenteric vein joining the splenic vein to form the portal vein, which then enters the liver. The hepatic portal vein tributaries drain the gastrointestinal tract, gall bladder, and spleen. The portal vein empties into sinusoids (small blood vessels) in the liver.

The portal vein, unlike other veins in the body, both starts and ends with capillaries. The significance of this is that digested foodstuffs in the alimentary canal are absorbed into the capillaries which go to make up the portal vein and are carried by it to the liver. In order that these nutrients and materials can come in contact with the individual liver cells for further chemical action or storage, it is necessary for the blood to pass through a second set of capillaries. **The interchange of substances between blood and tissues can take place only through capillaries.** The portal vein itself is quite short, approximately 7.5cm (3 inches), and is positioned just behind the pancreas whence it passes upwards, behind the pylorus, to reach the portal fissure of the liver.

The **nervous system** is composed of all the nerves in the body. The function of nerve tissue is to: receive stimuli, transmit to nerve centres, and to initiate a response. The central nervous system consists of the brain and spinal cord and serves as the collection point of nerve impulses. The peripheral nervous system includes all the nerves not in the brain or spinal cord and connects all parts of the body to the central nervous system. The peripheral (sensory) nervous system receives stimuli, the central nervous system interprets them, and then the peripheral (motor) nervous system initiates a response. (See Table 5a)

The **autonomic nervous system**, mostly motor nerves, controls functions of involuntary smooth muscles, cardiac muscles, and glands. This is the part of the nervous system that supplies the internal organs, including the blood vessels, stomach, intestine, liver, kidneys, bladder, genitals, lungs, pupils and muscles of the eyes, and heart and sweat, salivary, and digestive glands. The autonomic nervous system has two main divisions: the **sympathetic and the parasympathetic.**

After the autonomic nervous system receives information about the body and external environment, it responds by stimulating body processes, usually through the sympathetic system, or inhibiting them, usually through the parasympathetic system. The sympathetic system activates and prepares the body for vigorous muscular activity, stress, and emergencies (fight or flight) while the parasympathetic system lowers activity, operates during normal activities, permits digestion, and conservation of energy, that is, brings the body back to rest. **These systems generally work in a balanced and reciprocal way.** For example: the sympathetic nervous system will reduce saliva production; increase heart rate and dilate coronary arteries; relax bronchial muscle and dilates bronchi; reduces stomach peristalsis; reduce small intestine motility; reduce large intestine motility; increase liver conversion of glycogen to glucose; decrease the secretion of urine by the kidneys; relax the bladder wall and closes sphincter; will increases sweating; and encourages secretion of adrenalin.

The parasympathetic nervous system will increase saliva production; decrease dry mouth; decrease heart rate; constrict bronchial muscle; increase secretion of gastric juice and stomach motility; increase digestion in small intestine; increase motility in large intestine; constrict liver; increase urine secretion; decrease release of adrenalin; contract wall of bladder, and relax sphincter.

So, in summary, general stimulation of the parasympathetic nervous system promotes vegetative (unconscious functions) of the body. Stimulation of the parasympathetic and inhibition of the sympathetic have the same overall effects.

Additional functions associated with the colon, of the parasympathetic nervous system, are as follows:

- Peristaltic contraction will increase emptying of the gall bladder, stomach, and small intestine.

- Relaxation of sphincter muscles will facilitate emptying into the colon.

- Peristaltic contraction of the colon wall and sphincter muscles will facilitate defecation.

As we have discussed, mass **peristaltic movements** push faecal material from the sigmoid colon into the rectum. The distension of the rectal wall initiates a reflex for defecation, the emptying of the rectum. Motor impulses travel along parasympathetic nerves back to the descending colon, sigmoid colon, rectum, and anus.

Contraction of the longitudinal rectal muscles shortens the rectum and thus increases the pressure inside of it. This pressure, along with our voluntary contractions of our diaphragm and abdominal muscles (increasing pressure inside the abdomen) forces the anal sphincter open and the faeces are expelled through the anus.

The external sphincter is voluntarily controlled. If and when it is relaxed defecation happens, and if and when voluntarily constricted defecation can be postponed.

Discussion with patients about frequency of elimination and the form of faecal matter and stools is an essential aspect of colon hydrotherapy. Stool consistency can vary between hard lumps to very loose and mushy. This will depend upon, for example, the contents of a meal, how long stools have been in the colon, and how much water has been absorbed by them in the process.

The stool can be assessed and classified by:

a) Colon Transit Time. It is postulated by some colon hydrotherapists that the number of bowel movements per day, for the healthy person, will equal the number of meals eaten, that is, two or three times. Given that there is a wide range of 'normal' bowel function between different people it is also argued that there is probably no right or wrong answer. The important point is that stools are passed without excessive urgency; with minimal effort and without straining; without the use of laxatives; are formed into soft and smooth sausage shapes, and are passed, as regularly as possible, and for many persons, daily. Straining means the stool has insufficient moisture or bulk necessary to build momentum for easy evacuation.

b) Size, Shape, and Texture. Faeces consist of water, inorganic salts, sloughed-off epithelial cells from the mucosa of gastrointestinal tract, bacteria, products of bacterial decomposition, and undigested parts of food. (Tortora and Anagnostakos, 1990). Faeces form between 6 to 10% of the food ingested. Faeces are normally a semi-solid mass, with a mucous coating. Water, even after the absorption that takes place in the colon, still forms approximately 65% the total bulk of the faeces, with bacteria around a further 30%. The composition of the stool is also dependent on the amount of fat consumed. Normal stool contains around 1% fat. The passage of abnormally increased amounts of fat in faeces due to reduced absorption by the small intestine (or the consumption of high amounts of fat) is a condition known as 'steatorrhoea'. If the problem is chronic it may be due to a lack of enzymes being produced by the pancreas. A soft fibre-less stool becomes difficult for the bowel to move along.

The **Bristol Stool Chart** or the Bristol Stool Scale is a medical aid designed to classify the faeces form into seven groups or types. It was developed by K W Heaton and S J Lewis at the University of Bristol and was first published in the Scandinavian Journal of Gastroenterology in 1997. The form of the stool depends on the time it spends in the colon. The seven types of stool are described as follows:

Type 1: Separate hard lumps, like nuts and are hard to pass.

Type 2: Sausage-shaped, but lumpy.

Type 3: Like a sausage but with cracks on the surface.

Type 4: Like a sausage or snake, smooth and soft.

Type 5: Soft blobs with clear-cut edges, and passed easily.

Type 6: Fluffy, with ragged edges, a mushy stool.

Type 7: Watery, with no solid pieces, entirely liquid.

Types 1 and 2 above indicate constipation; caused by

dehydrating foods and drinks, for example, processed foods high in sugar and salt; dehydrating coffee and alcohol. Also, excessive transit time often linked to lack of fruit, vegetables, and wholegrain in the diet and insufficient intake of water and other pathological causes of constipation. As a consequence these high- density stools will quickly sink in water. Hard pellet stools can also be a sign of adrenal exhaustion, and emotional blockage. (See 'Indications for Colon Hydrotherapy' section).

Types 3 and 4 being the 'ideal stools' especially the latter, as these are appropriately formed, are comfortable and easy to pass.

Types 5 to 7 are tending towards diarrhoea (or are actual diarrhoea) caused by pathogens, irritation, inflammation, stress, drugs, laxatives, and other pathological causes. The body is certainly telling us something is wrong and must never be ignored. (See 'Indications for Colon Hydrotherapy' section).

Mucous in the stools is indicative of an irritated colon caused by lack of digestive enzymes, for example, poor carbohydrate digestion; a diet high in mucous-forming foods, for example, wheat and dairy (leading to mucoidal plaque); pathological disorders, for example, ulcerative colitis or IBS; or pathogens, for example, parasites.

The colon will produce excessive mucous mostly for its own protection, or in order to increase the elimination of toxins and waste.

Chronic constipation, mucous-forming diets, and excessive meat in the diet, leads to the bowel becoming **impacted.** This in turn leads to a **narrowed passage** for stool elimination and therefore is one of the causes of the formation of **narrow stools,** which may also be indicative of a spastic colon. This narrowing means that sometimes bowel movements/stools become ribbon like. The colon will often feel sore. Other causes of narrow and ribbon-like stools include: lack of fibre, stress, allergies, and structural/functional factors.

Undigested foodstuff in the stools may be indicative of poorly chewed food, lack of digestive enzymes, insufficient friendly bacteria and pH being too alkaline thus causing constipation to occur. One of the main causes of pH above 7 is undigested protein as a of poor digestion and intestinal flora imbalance.

c) Colour. Faeces are normally coloured brown by stercobilin, a pigment derived from the bilirubin and biliverdin of the bile. If stools are **black** this could be indicative of bleeding in the gastrointestinal tract, the ingestion of iron, dark berries, charcoal (in the treatment of excess acid in the stomach). If bleeding occurs lower down in the gastrointestinal tract, for example due to haemorrhoids, stools will become mixed with **bright red** blood.

For Patients who, for example, develop a stone that blocks the common bile duct, stools will be **pale or 'white'** in colour. Pale stools can also be caused by low-fibre diets, high in fat and processed foods, anaemia, and liver dysfunction. A very **dark brown** stool may suggest liver dysfunction or as the result, for example, of excess chlorophyll as in a diet rich in leafy vegetables. A **'green' stool** is considered to result from rapid transit of faeces through the colon. A **'clay-like'** appearance is considered to result from a lack of bilirubin. Artificial food colouring in processed foods can, if eaten in sufficient quantity, colour faeces.

When the colon has a beneficial balance of bacteria in the colon pathogenic bacteria will be eliminated. When stools are dry, dark brown, too solidly formed, or too loose, and especially if there is a putrid odour, these are clear signs of a putrefactive, alkaline-producing colon flora.

d) Odour. In a healthy person, stools will be only slightly fetid. The distinctive odour of faeces is due to bacterial action producing sulphur-containing compounds such as skatole and indole, as well as the inorganic gas hydrogen sulphide.

The consumption of foods rich in spices may result in the spices being undigested and therefore adding to the odour of the faeces. Moreover, the consumption of high levels of fat in the diet is often the cause of offensive-smelling stools, which may look greasy, are soft, and often difficult to flush away, as they tend to stick to the sides of the toilet bowl.

Greasy stools may also result from insufficient bile so that fats are not being properly broken down. (It is known that patients suffering from hepatitis and cirrhosis pass particularly odoriferous stools).

Excessively offensive stools caused by the presence of toxins can be indicators of disease as the body attempts to respond to the presence of toxins by producing neutrophil leukocytes, (an important defense against infection). These release active oxygen in an attempt to neutralize the damage to organs that can be caused by these waste products.

However, when an excessive amount of such active oxygen is produced it can damage healthy cells, as well as neutralize toxins. The Patient can minimize the harmful effect by addressing underlying causes and supplementing diet with vitamin E, given its role in protecting cells and tissues against oxidation and injury from unstable molecules and pollution. Sulphur-containing compounds (for example, indole and skatole) are also responsible for flatulence.

e) Gas. (Also see Bloating and Gas in section on Indications for Colon Hydrotherapy Treatment). Gas results naturally as a bi-product of metabolism. In the healthy person this will cause no bloating and is odourless. In the colonic tube this will appear as a few medium-sized bubbles and be without any associated pain. However, in treatment Patients may also show:

Bloating, with little wind being passed, (showing small bubbles, large wind pockets in the colonic tube, and including difficulties in releasing), is caused by spasms, poor digestion, and fermenting bowel flora.

Bloating, with a lot of wind being passed, (showing no difficulties in releasing, but showing constant small bubbles in the colonic tube, and pain), is caused by fermentation, due to bad digestion, and fermenting bowel flora.

No bloating but excessive amounts of wind being passed, (showing

162

medium-sized bubbles with occasional larger pockets in the colonic tube, and with no pain), caused by poor protein breakdown and putrefaction; gobbling down food; excessive carbon dioxide from bacterial breathing. (Scottish School of Colonic Hydrotherapy, 2007).

In order to begin to address gas and bloating it is advised to eat smaller quantities of food, and to chew food thoroughly, thus aiding the digestive enzymes in breaking food down. Also, avoid drinking with meals.

Regular bowel movement activity promotes health. An underactive bowel movement increases the burden on the other organs of elimination

Remember: it is very important to allow sufficient time for release. It is recommended when sitting upon the toilet to use a small stool upon which to place your feet and thus raise the knees. This is how we are designed to evacuate, in a **squatting posture,** over a hole in the ground, not sitting upon a porcelain toilet!

Colon hydrotherapy is the first line of defence against the accumulation of waste and faeces and is the best means of maintaining a clean colon. This in turn helps keep the **appendix** in good working order, thus facilitating its function regarding the secretion of germicidal fluid into the caecum to combat potentially harmful matter.

The Urinary System

The urinary system is formed by the following structures:

- The **kidneys** - the excretory glands.
- The **ureters** - the ducts of the kidneys.
- The **bladder** - the urinary reservoir.
- The **urethra** - the channel to the exterior.

The kidneys lie embedded in perinephric fat (the prefix peri- denoting around or enclosing), on the posterior abdominal wall, but are situated behind the peritoneum. The right kidney is actually slightly lower in

163

position than the left.

The **primary function of the kidneys** is to help in keeping the composition of the blood constant by excreting either abnormal constituents or the excess of normally present substances. The entire volume of blood in the body is filtered by the kidneys approximately 60 times a day. In performing this function they maintain fluid and electrolyte balance and ensure:

- The **excretion of water**, a certain quantity of water only is necessary to maintain blood and tissue fluids.

- The **excretion of the end-products of protein metabolism**; urea is the most important of these end-products and forms half of the total of the solid constituents of the urine (96% water and 4% solids). It is formed in the liver by the removal of the nitrogen-containing fraction of the aminoacids.

- The **excretion of salts**, which are the chlorides, phosphates, and sulphates and oxalates of sodium, potassium, and calcium. Salts may be acid, neutral, or alkaline and it is one of the essential functions of kidneys to keep a very slightly alkaline blood pH constant. One of the most important salts circulating in the blood is sodium bicarbonate, an alkali, which in the presence of acids sets free carbonic acid and becomes a neutral salt. In this way any excess acid is neutralized.

- The **excretion of drugs, toxins, and chemical substances** that may be harmful, and in doing so, return the substances that the body requires and eliminate in the urine the remainder. The formation of urine involves three processes:

Filtration. This process takes place in the Malpighian bodies, blood capilliaries of the glomerulus, site of primary filtration, and its surrounding Bowman's capsule. The blood pressure forces water and dissolved substances through the endothelial walls of the capilliaries and on through the filtration slits of the adjoining wall of the glomerular, Bowman's capsule. The resulting fluid is called **filtrate**. The amount of filtrate that flows out of all the renal corpuscles of both kidneys every minute is called the glomerular filtration rate (GFR). In the normal adult, this rate is about 125ml/minute. That is about 180l (48 gallons) a day. (You will remember that the entire body contains around 45l of blood (10 gallons) which is pumped by the heart throughout the whole body at the rate of around 90l a day, with a healthy heart striking around 100,000 beats daily in order to maintain this twice daily movement and filtration of the system!

Secretion. This process is performed by the cells of the epithelium lining the convoluted tubules. These cells select either abnormal substances or normal substances from the blood when their concentration exceeds their threshold value and passes them into the lumen of the tubules. As we know it is very important for the body to maintain blood glucose at a constant level. If unduly low, hypoglycaemia occurs, or if excessively high, hyperglycaemia occurs. Normally, no sugar is excreted by the kidneys. Unless very excessive quantities are taken the body is able to use it and convert it into carbon dioxide and water and to store the excess as glycogen in the liver. In diabetes, the deficiency of insulin makes it impossible for the tissues to utilize sugar, hence it tends to accumulate in the blood and the blood sugar rises. In order to counteract this, the kidneys begin to excrete sugar in an attempt to reduce blood sugar to normal.

Absorption. If all the fluid and salts passing from the glomeruli into the tubules by the process of filtration were allowed to pass to the exterior in the urine there would be a serious loss of valuable material from the body and blood composition would be affected. In order to prevent this, some of the water and salts are re-absorbed into the circulation by the kidney cells, especially those in the loop of Henle.

Urine passes via the collecting tubules into the pelvis of the kidney, the expanded upper part of **the ureter,** and then down the ureter, a tube, by the peristaltic action of its walls. The ureter is around 25cm in length, (10 inches). The lower portion of the ureter is called the pelvic part and, in the female, is close to the side of the cervix of the uterus.

The bladder, or reservoir in which urine is received, lies in front of the rectum in the male, but in the female is separated from the rectum by the uterus and vagina. The bladder can contain 700 to 800ml of urine. When the amount exceeds 200 to 400ml the **micturition reflex**, desire to expel urine, is initiated. The will can control the act and, if necessary postpone emptying. The volume of urine eliminated per day in the normal adult varies between 1,000 to 2,000ml (2 to 4 pints). The lowest part of the bladder is called the base and surrounds the opening of the urethra.

The urethra is the canal conveying the urine from the bladder to the exterior. As it leaves the bladder it is surrounded by a sphincter muscle.

Urine is slightly acidic, but depending upon the internal environment and varying pathological conditions, the characteristics of urine may change dramatically. Urine analysis tells us much about the state of the body.

The prostate gland is located between the neck of the urinary bladder and the rectum indicating the importance of avoiding inflammation and infection by insuring the system is 'flushed', that is, drinking lots of water.

A healthy urinary system is essential to good health. Bacteria can infect an unhealthy urinary tract, which may lead to prolonged illness and fever. In patients with poor kidney health it is likely that uric acid crystals will form in the joints, and cause gout, and in other parts of the body such accumulation is called acidosis. However, the most familiar kidney problem is kidney stones. These stones, crystallized mineral deposits, are very painful when evacuated through urination, and if sufficiently large can block the urinary flow.

Drinking tea made from Cleaver's Herb (also known as Goose Grass) will help dissolve kidney stones (and gall stones), is a cleansing diuretic, and is used to counter toxic conditions. It can be taken in quite large quantities, especially if taken as a tea brewed from the freshly gathered herb, and is also available as a tincture.

The Lungs

The lungs occupy the greater part of the thoracic cavity. The right lung has three lobes: upper, middle and lower; and the left two lobes, upper and lower (it is thought to allow for the accommodation of the heart). The apex rises into the root of the neck for about 2.5cm above the clavicle. The base is concave and is related to the upper surface of the diaphragm.

The expansion of the lungs causes air to be sucked in through the upper air passages and trachea. With expiration the capacity of the thorax returns to its former size and air is expelled from the lungs. **Internal respiration** occurs as oxygen is transferred from the blood to the tissues of the body that at the same time give up carbon dioxide and other waste gases for **elimination through expiration.** Inhalation through the nose means that mucous membrane warms, moisten, and traps dirt and dust as air passes down the throat and into the trachea.

Atmospheric air is a mixture of gases, approximately: oxygen (20%), carbon dioxide (0.04%) and nitrogen (79%). Expired air contains 16% oxygen, 4% carbon dioxide, and 79% nitrogen, and of course water vapour and heat.

Normal respiration in adults is 16 to 18 breaths per minute. Ordinarily, respiration is an automatic act under the unconscious control of the nervous system. The respiratory system is especially sensitive to the amount of carbon dioxide (carbonic acid) in the blood. If the amount rises (say during muscular exercise), impulses are sent out to the respiratory muscles to produce deeper and quicker breathing in order that carbon dioxide is excreted more rapidly and thus lower the amount in the blood to its normal level.

If the lungs are clogged with toxins they will no longer be strong enough to eliminate properly. Therefore all the organs and tissues of the body will be affected. Levels of carbonic acid in the bloodstream will be increased which in turn reduces oxygenation. Poor respiration is associated with allergies, asthma, lymph congestion, catarrhal problems, fatigue, acidity throughout the body, and lower metabolism.

When the lungs are healthy they can eliminate as much as 1kg of waste materials daily.

Catarrh (phlegm and mucous) is **symptomatic of imbalances** in the body. It is often the first symptom to appear and is often a clear indication of an excess of acids and mucous due to inflammation. Catarrh is produced as a protection from irritants, is made by goblet cells in the mucous membrane linings, and acts as a lubricant. When germs and toxins enter the body they are excreted as catarrh flowing mucous. Catarrh can also occur in Patient's who have certain allergies or food sensitivities. We know that certain foods may be the direct cause of illness, phlegm, catarrh, for example: excess dairy, refined carbohydrates, sugar, and meat.

The respiratory membranes are an active and receptive surface, and like the intestines, have the same primary cellular structure as the skin. Inhalation of steam is often used to stimulate the mucous membranes of the nose and sinuses, and to mobilize catarrhal secretions. Using aromatic oils such as wintergreen, eucalyptus, and clove, or with oils being rubbed on the chest, in order to increase the stimulus is often recommended. (Turner R N, 2000)

Breathing is Life. Get rid of catarrh by cleansing the system. The following is a tested cleansing diet for the removal of catarrh. Initially, follow the diet for up to five days and increase for a further five days as appropriate:

Morning: Oranges, or orange and lemon juice, or grapefruit. (No sugar).

Midday: Raw salad consisting of any vegetable (in season if possible). Use a dressing of garlic and cold-pressed virgin olive oil. Followed by a dessert of raisins, prunes (soaked), figs, or dates.

Evening: Raw salad or one or two vegetables steamed in their own juice, such as spinach, cauliflower, cabbage, carrots, turnips, etc.

Finish with a few nuts or sweet fruit such as apples, pears, plums, or cherries. No drinks other than filtered water. Nothing should be added to the above list. If bread, potatoes, or other starchy food are taken the effect of the diet will be lost. (See also section on Cleansing and Detoxification Diets).

It is essential that we each do our best to find opportunities to breathe fresh, clean air. For those of us living in towns or polluted cities it becomes even more critical. A brisk, early morning walk, when the air is fresher, is recommended. There is a history of different breathing patterns or systems available to us from those taught through: Hatha Yoga, Tai-chi, Qui-Gong, and more recently, Buteyko breathing exercises. The primary objective is the one of exercising the lungs through physical exercise, being mindful of the flow of breath, and consciously exhaling impurities and toxins.

Take time each day to undertake a series of 10 complete breaths by breathing deeply into the abdomen allowing the abdomen to rise, hold briefly (do not exhale), and breathe in again and consciously take air deep into the lungs and up into the area of the clavicles, now feeling the whole of the abdomen and lungs are completely full of air, hold the breath again for a count of three or four. Exhale from the top of the lungs, down through the respiratory system, and emptying out the bottom of the lungs and base of the stomach as if emptying a vessel of fluid, cleansing as we exhale. With eyes closed allow the 'in and out' breath to 'massage' every organ, tissue, and cell of the body. As oxygen is invigorating it is of no surprise that this series of 'complete breathing exercises' will stimulate, cleanse, and energise the whole body.

According to the ancient yoga texts, (yoga means the union of the individual self with the universal self) the practice of 'Pranayama' is a conscious prolongation of inhalation, retention, and exhalation. Inhalation is the act of receiving energy in the form of breath. Retention is when the breath is held in order to savour (utilize) that energy. When exhaling, all thoughts and emotions are emptied with the breath. While the lungs are empty, one surrenders the individual energy, 'I', to the primeval (universal) energy. This practise develops

169

a steady mind, sound judgement, health, balance, release of all tensions, and stimulates an inner awareness. (Iyengar B K S, 1983).

The Skin

The skin is the body's largest organ and has the following parts:

The **epidermis** or outer layer, consists of keratinocytes having migrated from the deeper layers (the basal layer where basal cells continuously divide, forming keratinocytes) of the epidermis and are finally and continuously shed from the surface of the skin. The epidermis also prevents the entry of foreign substances and bacteria.

The **dermis** or inner layer containing:

sweat glands, all over the body but most abundantly in the palms of the hands, soles of feet, and on the forehead, consisting of a coiled tube with an opening on the surface by a pore, secretion of sweat is controlled by the action of the sympathetic nerves and is 99% water, sodium chloride, and minute quantities of other waste products;

sebaceous glands, which secrete sebum to keep skin supple and the hairs from becoming brittle;

nerve endings, which are mainly sensory;

blood vessels and capillaries, and

lymph glands.

The **appendages:** nails and hair are composed mainly of the protein keratin. The health of hair, scalp, and nails depends on a good
balance of minerals and vitamins. The oils of bergamot and lavender mixed in equal quantities and added to a carrier oil can be an effective treatment for dandruff.

Primary Functions of the Skin:

- Forms a protective covering for the body.

- Contains the end-organs of the sensory nerves (pain, touch, and temperature).

- Secretes sebum.

- Is capable of absorbing small amounts of oily substances.

- Gives origin to hair and nails.

- Contains ergosterol, a substance converted into vitamin D by the action of sunlight which plays an important role in the metabolism of calcium and proper absorption of calcium from the intestine.

- By secreting sweat the skin acts as an excretory organ, removing waste products, water and salts; plays an important part in the regulation of body temperature

When healthy, the **temperature** of the body is maintained at an average level of 37 degrees centigrade (98.4 degrees fahrenheit), but shows slight variations during the day, being a little lower in the early morning.

Remember: heat production is produced by the chemical processes of metabolism, and is greatly increased by muscular exercise. Heat is principally lost through the skin. The pituitary gland (posterior lobe) basically controls body temperature and regulation of water. When the body is hot the pores open, when cold the pores close.

A full-body massage has similar effects upon the skin as cold and hot water treatment. It accelerates the circulation, draws blood to the surface, opens and relaxes the pores, promotes elimination, and intensifies the latent electromagnetic energies in the body of the Patient. Furthermore, it is now common knowledge that a head, neck, face, and shoulder massage, can be a real stressbuster: relaxing the muscles and skin and encourages the elimination of toxins that have accumulated in the mind and the body!

Moreover, always remember the value of **exercise and fresh air**, hot then cold showers, a **friction bath** (the skin being rubbed with a rough towel followed by a cold shower), and skin brushing.

Skin brushing is another excellent way to detoxify the skin and promote circulation. Ensure Patients are advised to avoid rashes, infections, and cuts. Use a brush made from natural fibres and begin each day by brushing the bottoms of the feet up and down and then from side to side about six times, respectively. (The treatment of brushing the bottoms of the feet will also help every organ of the body, as will reflexology). Then brush from the tops of the feet up and down and from side to side. Brush up the legs towards the knees and then from the knees to the hips. Brush the buttocks in a circular motion and then brush the abdomen in a circular motion. Then brush up to the heart.

Women (and men) are advised to brush the breast area gently and avoid brushing the nipples. Brush the upper part of the chest downwards toward the heart. Brush the palms of the hands and tops of the hands up and down and from side to side. Brush arms up toward the heart and brush the back with up and down strokes. Use a smaller and softer brush for the face and neck. Brush from the throat up toward the face and then brush the skin of the face from the jaw up. For the forehead, brush from side to side.

When this routine is completed, follow up with a relaxing shower or bath. Rinse brushes in warm water and a natural liquid soap once a week and allow them to dry before using again. (Jensen E, 2005).

Linseed oil and olive oil are helpful in keeping the skin pliable and moist. Vitamin A, silicon, and zinc help build the skin. Vitamin C, with bioflavonoids, tightens connective tissue and prevents varicose veins. (Bioflavonoids increase the strength of the capillaries and help to regulate permeability. Sources include: citrus fruits, apricots, broccoli, and tomatoes). Dark-green leafy vegetables are excellent foods to help cleanse the skin.

Avoid cosmetics and deodorants that contain aluminium (which can be toxic and is also found in refined foods, in processed cheese as an emulsifier, in aluminium pots and pans, and in common table salt). Choose soaps, oils, lotions, and deodorants that are made with natural ingredients.

Specific **essential oils**, blends of essential oils, and massage oils are antimicrobial, antifungal, and antiyeast. They also have highly oxygenating molecules and therefore deliver oxygen to cells and help the immune system fight off the ravages of disease. When essential oils are used for massage they are mixed with 'carrier' oils, for example, unperfumed vegetable oil, sweet almond oil, and grapeseed oil.

The essential oils of **fennel, juniper, and rose** contain detoxifying qualities. Essential oils like **geranium, lavender, and sandalwood** have a balancing effect on sebum (the natural lubricant of the skin), and regular massage will increase the circulation in the blood vessels that feed the growing layer of skin, thus improving the health, vitality, and nourishment of the skin.

Note: **aloe vera** is also an important healer for skin-related concerns, including the colon mucosa. It is detoxifying, encourages beneficial bacteria, is antiviral, and enhances the immune system.

We have discussed above the general benefits of massage. Massage also provides a boost to the lymphatic system and its function concerning the removal of toxins clogging the tissues, including the dermis.

The Lymphatic System

The lymphatic system is a subsidiary or second circulatory system, which drains the **tissue fluids** that act as a sort of 'halfway house' between the blood on the one hand and the tissues on the other. All **interchange of nourishment and waste products** takes place through the medium of the tissue fluid, which passes into narrow vessels, the lymphatic vessels.

Strictly speaking, lymph is the name given to the tissue fluid when it has passed into the lymphatic vessels. The smaller vessels eventually converge into two large ducts. The most important of these is the **thoracic duct.**

This duct is about 36cm (15 inches) long and starts as a dilated sac, the **cisterna chyli,** into which the lymph vessels from the lower limbs and the contents of the abdominal cavity, particularly the intestines, empty their lymph. It is situated in front of the upper lumbar vertebrae (L2) on the right of the abdominal aorta.

The **lymphatics of the intestines** are of particular importance, because all digested fat is absorbed through them. It is through the minute projections from the mucous membrane of the intestine (the villi) each containing a small lymphatic vessel (the lacteal) into which the digested fat (chyle) is absorbed and will ultimately pass to the cisterna chyli.

The **lymphatic glands**, generally occurring in groups on the course of the lymphatic vessels, act as a filter for the lymph. **Among the most important** are: the cervical (situated in the neck) **axillary** (situated in the arm pit) and **inguinal** (situated in the groin). Deeper lymph glands are the **iliac** (situated in the right iliac fossa, a concave depression on the inside of the pelvis that provides space for the vermiform appendix); **lumbar** (close to the lumbar vertebrae); **the thoracic** (at the root of the lungs); **mesenteric** (situated in the mesentery, a double layer of peritoneum, of the intestines); and the **portal** (in the portal fissure of the liver).

Therefore, the **lymph system primarily works with the elimination systems** by serving as a 'rubbish' collector by carrying metabolic by-products and accumulated cellular waste from the tissues to the elimination organs.

When the lymph stream is over burdened, the impurity will finally get to the joints and other parts of the body in the form of uric acid and catarrh. This can cause rheumatic problems or it can carry toxic waste from the colon to the other tissues in the body causing toxaemia, infections, inflammation, aches, and pains.

An overload of catarrh and bacteria cause the lymph glands to become painful and swollen. Some patients will have an inherently weak lymph system and hold water in their tissues more than others and show puffiness in their face, hands, and feet.

In addition to colon hydrotherapy, some Practitioners perform lymph-drainage therapy which uses light touch to detect the quality of the lymph flow and to stimulate lymph and interstitial fluid circulation. This modality encourages detoxification, regeneration of tissues, and a **healthy immune system.**

Immunity is the body's capability to repel foreign substances and cells. Lymph organs, in addition to lymph glands, include bone marrow, the spleen, and thymus. Bone marrow produces lymphocytes and these are primarily responsible for immunity, circulating antibodies, and T-lymphocytes. The thymus gland secretes the hormone, thymosin, which causes pre-T cells to mature into T cells. The spleen serves as a reservoir for blood, and filters the blood and lymph fluid that flows through it.

So, as can be seen, the lymph system is a major part of a properly functioning immune system. Whilst the cardio-vascular system utilizes the heart as a pump to push blood through the body the lymphatic circulation is dependent upon breathing and exercise.

Therefore, the lymph system must be kept clean and free flowing. The body is composed of 75 to 80% distilled water. Plenty of fresh clean water is essential for the flow of the lymph. Also, in order to prevent lymphatic congestion, Practitioners are advised to recommend to their Patients, as appropriate, brisk walks, taking deep breaths, and swinging the arms, thus actively improving circulation. Remember, foods that can easily clog the lymphatic system are wheat and dairy products.

Cleansing and Detoxification Diets

The primary way of maintaining a relatively cleansed body is to combine colon hydrotherapy with a diet of organically grown fruits, vegetables, fresh fruit juices and vegetable juices, filtered or distilled warm water, and herbal teas. Such a diet, as noted earlier, requires minimal digestion and therefore more energy will be available for the process of elimination and far fewer unwanted toxins are consumed.

Cleansing and detoxification diets should leave the Patient feeling **cleansed and refreshed.** Such diets will help prepare the Patient for other dietary and lifestyle changes that the Patient may wish to make. Such diets can be transforming. The **goals are best summarized as:**

- Enabling the Patient to recognize inappropriate and damaging eating habits.

- Enabling the Patient to eliminate the burden of stimulants.

- Enabling the Patient to eliminate toxins.

- Achieve some weight loss

- Help the Patient clear their mind.

- Enable the Patient to establish for themselves a vitalized and refreshed body.

Contraindications for all cleansing diets include: Patients with anaemia, severe nutritional deficiency, diabetes, low blood-sugar levels, low blood pressure, pregnancy and lactation, liver and kidney disease, terminal illness, and for frail elderly people. Patients who are on prescription drugs should consult their Doctor before trying a cleansing programme. Patients with a nutritional deficiency are recommended to build up first, prior to starting any 'detox' regime.

We know that colon hydrotherapy will multiply the effectiveness of any cleanse programme (or maintenance regime) and in most cases should be the first stage in the cleansing process.

We know that diet directly influences health and therefore is something we are able to control, to a greater degree than other factors, for example, genetic inheritance or environmental pollutants. Physical stimuli, such as colon hydrotherapy, deep breathing, and moderate exercise, are all considered to be essential adjuncts to cleansing because they improve circulation and therefore the eliminative functions of the lungs, skin, and colon.

Remember that it is **unbeneficial to combine fruit and vegetables** at the same meal. Fruit does not combine well with other foods and this factor also applies to juices. Fruit ferments rapidly and takes around 30 minutes to pass through the stomach, whereas concentrated protein takes up to two to three hours. So eat fruit 30 minutes before a meal or not less than a couple of hours at least afterwards.

The length of time of a cleansing diet varies, although around five to 10 days is usual. The specific programme and the Patient's experience and needs will be the determining factors. The objective of the Practitioner is to support the Patient in a cleanse/detox routine that is relevant to their health needs and, for them, is something that is meaningful and achievable.

The benefits of using a cleansing diet are: **relief of pain, removal of toxins, and clearing of the mind.** Cleansing is always indicated for arthritis and mucous congestion. Cleansing will strip away the build-up of acid and ureas responsible for inflammation. Also, use fasting and cleansing diets for overweight.

In addition to the kidneys and bowel, elimination is likely to occur from other orifices – the nose, ears, mouth, and the skin. In fact, the skin (sometimes called the third kidney), is the largest organ of elimination. The skin is the barometer of health, reflecting many conditions that come from within: rashes, boils, and swellings. The skin shows our age, hygiene, circulation, digestion, and the effects of detoxification.

The possible side effects during a given fast or cleansing process may include: experiencing some physical and mental discomfort with feelings of irritability and impatience; obviously some hunger pangs; the Patient may also feel cold, develop a furred, white-coated tongue (a sign of the body eliminating toxins) halitosis, heightened body odour, constipation or diarrhoea, light-headedness, changes in sleeping patterns, headaches, and dizziness.

Some Practitioners believe that by working with the cycle of the moon, cleansing and detoxification programmes become more efficient. The period from a full moon to the next new moon is known as the waning phase and it is when our body energy levels rise and a natural detoxification cycle is entered. Therefore, any cleansing regime is said to be far more beneficial when the moon is waning.

Cleansing is different for everyone. Some Patients feel more energetic and active during their cleansing, for others, not until they have completed their cleansing diet. Remember, it is the body's wisdom that is working on those areas of the body that require help to regain optimum health. Discomfort associated with cleansing is usually only temporary and from it the Patient will derive more energy, vitality, and improved health.

It is recommended to come off any fast or cleanse **slowly.** It is advised, during the day following the end of the fast or cleansing programme that the Patient commences with fresh fruit salad, lightly steamed vegetables, or brown rice, organic yogurt, and plenty of warm water. Chewing foods slowly, so they are more easily digested, is important, as is the avoidance of heavy meals or over eating.

Fasting

Fasting is one of the most profound cleansing processes a person can undertake. **Fasting is a natural remedy.** (Remember to ensure there are no contraindications)

Fasting, like all cleansing and detoxification programmes and diets, is about clearing the body of congestion, sluggishness, stagnation, toxicity found in the tissues, cells, and body systems. Toxicity, as we have discussed elsewhere, is caused by the intake of toxins (and internal production of toxins) or poor elimination. Fasting is an ancient and very beneficial practice. **Fasting is about the avoidance of solid foods and cleansing the whole system.**

178

Fasting is not always easy to accomplish, but like most things in life it becomes easier with practise. It is suggested that your Patient prepares for their fast (as with all dietary changes) several days before they commence. Eating smaller meals before they abstain is advisable as this will begin to signal their mind, stomach, and appetite that less food is acceptable.

The choice of programme is best viewed as being part of the treatment plan and therefore builds into it support from the therapist. The Patient may need to share their plan with those closest to them, will need to ensure they have all they need including the time and space for them in order to focus upon their fast, and be very clear about beginning and end times. To begin with, weekends may be the best time to start. Weekends are a time when it is more likely to avoid the pressures and strain of work and physical labour, especially as during the fast the Patient may feel some tiredness and weakness.

Whilst on a fast routine Patients are advised to go to bed before 10pm so as to help their body cleanse itself during the natural purification time, during sleep. The Practitioner will ensure the Patient is clear, in their own mind, about why they are doing the fast and what it is they aim to achieve. The question they need to ask of themselves is, "What am I seeking?" **The reason for their fast is their goal/s. Fasting is the process used to achieve that goal/s.** Keeping the goal in mind, especially when hunger or the refrigerator beckons, is helpful!

The Patient may wish to start with a one-day fast, and work towards a two-day and then a three-day fast, and then for a longer, extended fast. Fasting is a time for 'denying' the body of the comfort food brings, as well as specific lifestyle habits. Fasting is often a time for personal reflection, hence its transforming quality. There will of course be times during a fast when Patients will be saying to themselves, 'I have fasted long enough, now is the time for my fast to end'! This is why preparation and clarity of purpose is both necessary and helpful in achieving best results.

179

Detoxification can be, as suggested, transformative at many levels: physical, psychological, and spiritual (hence its association with religious observances). In order to help in the elimination of toxins, **fasts are supported by drinking lots of filtered water.**

A teaspoon of *psyllium* seed powder in the morning and evening mixed with warm water will hasten the elimination of toxins. Alfalfa tablets can also help with cleansing the system.

Even after a one-day fast the Patient is likely to experience a sense of achievement, feel uplifted, and their body will certainly have benefited. Many people build into their routines a day a week, a couple of days a month, or longer periods of fasting. As an alternative to a complete fast from solid foods you may wish to consider with your Patient the option of trying a juice fast.

Juice Fasting

Juice fasting, like abstaining from solid foods, is undertaking something that is very **powerful regarding the cleansing and healing of the body.** Juice fasting involves the intake for a specified period, typically for one to three days, or can be longer, of consuming raw fruit juice and vegetable juice and water only.

Fruit and vegetable juices are filled with healing and cleansing properties, are an excellent source of vitamins and antioxidants, and they enable the body to **gently and safely detoxify.** The natural sugars in juices provide energy, flavour, and will help the Patient maintain their motivation to complete their cleansing. Patients are advised to use in their juicer machines fresh fruits or vegetables. Buy organic produce if possible and always wash thoroughly. If the produce is not organic avoid including their skins. Off-the-shelf juice products are acceptable as long as they are 100% juice without sugar or other additives.

Remember to avoid any product, containing protein or fat, such as milk or soy-based drinks as these will restart the digestive cycle and the associated pangs of hunger.

The suggested fruit juices are apple, grapefruit, watermelon, cranberry, pineapple, and grape. The suggested vegetable juices are carrot, celery, cabbage, greens, spinach and beet. The Practitioner may wish to recommend 'green drinks' made from green leafy vegetables that are high in chlorophyll and are very cleansing. (Add spirulina, which is a form of chlorophyll).

Fruit juices are considered to be cleansers and are therefore best taken in the morning. Vegetable juices are seen as restorers or builders and are best taken in the afternoon. Combine with fruit teas and water inbetween. Springtime is thought by some Practitioners to be the best time of the year for juice fasting.

A litre or so of fruit-based juice in the morning to early afternoon, and the same amount of vegetable-based juice for the afternoon and evening would seem reasonable. Advise the Patient to sip their juice drinks throughout the day and not to forget to drink plenty of filtered water.

If the Patient is working, or away from their home, one option is to make a thermos flask of juice, one for fruit juice, one for vegetable juice.

Depending upon the Patient, it may be best to start with a **'one-day lemon detoxification programme'.**

The lemon has been treasured throughout history. It is one of nature's top sources of the mineral potassium that aids in normalizing blood pressure and regulating the body's water balance. Lemons are also high in **citric acid,** which is found naturally in citrus fruits and is essential for the energy-producing Krebs Cycle, to occur in all our cells.

As lemons contain 5 to 6% citric acid compared with oranges (1.5%), they are an acid fruit and therefore a **highly rated germicide.** Lemons are especially tonic and when toxicity exists in the liver, kidneys, lungs, skin, or bowels, they act as a **cleanser.** The lemon is also high in **ascorbic acid** (vitamin C).

In addition to the juice of the lemon, ascorbic acid is found in the albedo (the white, slightly bitter-tasting, inner portion of the outer peel) and the flavedo, the exterior peel, which contains the flavour-rich sacs, zest, released when shredded or sliced. Lemons are one of the world's richest sources of the antioxidant, pectin. As lemons are a natural cleanser and normaliser, this one-day programme will begin the detoxification process as well as the softening and loosening of stools in readiness for your colon hydrotherapy treatment. This is an especially excellent preparation for Patients suffering with chronic constipation.

- Wash thoroughly and then slice one lemon, add **one pint** of fil-tered water and place in a liquidizer, **using the complete lemon** including the skin and pips. **(Remember, to convert pints to litres, multiply by 0.568; litres to pints, multiply by 1.760)**
- Strain and discard the pulp and then add **five pints** of filtered water, now making a **total of six pints.**
- Start your detoxification at around 8am.
- Drink one average water glass of the mixture every 15 minutes for the first hour.
- Followed by one glass of the mixture every 45 minutes until the mixture has been consumed.

If you start at around 8am you will have completed the programme by 3 to 4pm and keep to water or herbal teas for remainder of the day.

As a possible alternative, the Patient may choose to visit a medical herbalist who may suggest, as part of a detoxification diet a tea based upon dandelion root, marigold flowers, milk-thistle seed, or nettle.

Parasite Cleanse

(See also the section on 'Indications Concerning Parasite

Infections').

In our earlier discussion, we noted that parasite infections are common and often associated with a broad range of diseases. If you think the Patient may have intestinal parasites, various tests can be authorized by the Patient's doctor and this will define which type of organism is causing problems. The Dr Hulda Clark, 'Parasite Cleanse' is recommended (see useful addresses). Various herbs and dietary supplements may also constitute a treatment plan.

You will see when you investigate the many 'parasite cleanse' formulas that the following herbs are used widely: garlic, cloves, goldenseal, black walnut hull, wormwood, wormseed, pumpkin seeds, and grapefruit seed extract. Each has its own unique properties. Some have antimicrobial and antiyeast properties, others have properties for expelling roundworms, hookworms, and tapeworms, others like goldenseal are considered to be active against the parasite *Giardia lamblia*. *Giardia* affects humans we know, but did you know that it is one of the most common parasites infecting cats and dogs! Dr Clark's parasite cleanse combines black walnut hull, common cloves, and wormwood (pregnant or breast-feeding women and infants should not take wormwood because of toxicity).

Practitioners may also suggest dietary options to support the intestinal parasite cleanse. Try eating raw garlic (or chop up a clove and swallow with a drink of water before a main meal); pineapple contains the enzyme bromelain which can help clear tapeworms; carrots are rich in beta carotene, a precursor for vitamin A, which is believed to increase the body's resistance to penetration by parasite larvae. (Wong C, 2007).

Remember to also advise the Patient about probiotics, such as *lactobacillus acidophilus* in order to help rebuild beneficial intestinal bacteria. A high-fibre diet will assist intestinal cleansing. Two dessert spoonfuls of linseeds soaked in water and taken in the morning is a valuable dietary supplement and will assist the cleansing process and is something worth continuing as a start to each day (even though the linseeds have been soaked prior to consumption, it is advisable to also drink one or two glasses of water afterwards).

Kidney Cleanse

Each day our **toxin-filtering kidneys** process about 227l of blood (400 pints) and manage to remove around 2.27l (4 pints) of waste and excess water. Without our kidneys waste products would simply build up in our blood. As a result of such toxic build-up and/or dietary neglect our kidneys become inflamed, infected, and develop stones or indeed fail altogether.

The kidneys regulate our pH balance, water, calcium, sodium, and potassium levels. Our kidneys help regulate blood pressure, stimulate the production of red blood cells, and also electrolyte formation. (When salt is dissolved, its elements, sodium and chloride, become important electrolytes which are responsible for transferring electrical energy within in the body). **Kidney damage usually takes place gradually and without symptoms.** If left untreated kidney disease can become irreversible.

There are many herbs, juices, and formulae that will help detoxify the urinary system. Ingredients may include: parsley, basil, celery, apple juice, black cherry concentrate, goldenrod tincture, and watermelon (which contains the highest concentration of water amongst all fruits, is rich in potassium salts, and is one of the safest and best diuretics).

What is essential in helping the kidneys to cleanse is to ensure a **liberal amount of clean filtered water** is consumed daily. The more water the Patient drinks the more toxins the body is able to expel as part of the following cleanse:

- Prepare by washing thoroughly one bunch of parsley, add just over half a pint of water, and boil for three minutes. When cool drain the parsley 'tea', drink half a cup, and place the remainder in a glass vessel and place in the refrigerator. This leaves approximately three half cups for the next three days. Repeat accordingly for a total of 20 days. Parsley acts as a diuretic and therefore is helpful in flushing the kidneys.

- Drink one glass of organic apple juice with 20 drops of dandelion, a root tincture, three times a day for 20 days. Apple pectin has a detoxifying quality. Dandelion has historically been used for kidney (and liver) problems and is also detoxifier.

- Include daily a therapeutic supplement of vitamin B6 (100 to 150mg) or combine with the other B complex vitamins. Vitamin B6 aids fluid balance regulation.

  Hydrangea root is recommended for dissolving kidney stones. The root also contains several alkaloids, many are naturally alkaline and have antioxidant and immune-supportive properties.

  Needless to say avoid, especially during your kidney cleanse, dairy produce, excessive protein, white flour, sugar products, meat, stimulants, rich foods, and overeating.

Liver Cleanse

Toxicity in your body is increased as a result of poor elimination through the colon, liver, kidneys, skin, and respiratory tract. **The liver is the most important detoxification organ** in your body and everyone needs to undertake cleansing as part of their healthcare routine. **Cleansing your liver will lead to a renewed sense of wellbeing** and your liver will feel rested, cleansed, and will function more effectively.

The following recipe will enable you to **flush your liver**. Drink the 'remedy' in place of your normal breakfast. Follow within 15 minutes with a 'detox-tea' or peppermint tea. No food should be eaten for at least one and a half hours after your drink. **Try for five mornings. Whatever you can manage your liver will appreciate.** Take a days rest and repeat for five days. You can strengthen the flush by increasing, proportionately, the amounts of garlic and ginger. Drink lots of clean filtered water and ensure a good fibre diet in order to facilitate regular bowel movement.

Whilst on your cleanse **avoid** all fried foods, dairy products (including eggs), alcohol, coffee, fizzy drinks, processed food, sugar products, and reduce to a minimum your meat consumption and avoid red meats completely. If possible, eat fresh, organically grown fruit and vegetables as these are **alkalising foods** and will help strip away the build-up of acids associated with toxicity.

Prepare your liver cleanse drink in the morning. Liquidise and drink slowly, on an empty stomach.

- 200ml (an average sized glass for water) of organic apple juice with half a squeezed lemon. (As an alternative you may choose pineapple, grape juice, beet, or carrot juice, but never mix fruit and vegetables together).

- Three tablespoons of extra virgin olive oil.

- One clove of organically grown garlic chopped prior to blending.

- A piece of fresh ginger to match size of garlic chopped prior to blending.

- A pinch or two of cayenne pepper.

- You may add a glass of filtered water if you wish.

- You may add a dessertspoonful of lecithin or linseed for fibre and sustenance.

Remember, drink plenty of filtered water, reduce stress as much as possible, and try to rest as much as you are able to. If you find it helpful, gently massage your stomach, from right to left. By day two you may experience symptoms of detoxification. Supplementary additions include **milk thistle**, a liver protector which contains antioxidant and anti-inflammatory substances; **burdock root**, also a liver cleanser and protector; dandelion root, good for liver repair, increases bile and is a laxative; **yellow dock** increases bile, reduces inflammation and mucous, and is a blood and liver cleanser.

A well-tested cleansing treatment, and favourite among many, is the easy to purchase **castor oil pack treatment**. This is an excellent all-round companion. Absorption through the skin and into the lymphatic system enhances immunity, helps balance the sympathetic and parasympathetic nervous system, disperses congestion and hardened mucous, and helps to release blockages in the bowel pockets.

Castor oil packs can be used anywhere on the body where there is inflammation or congestion, can be used as part of a cleansing programme, and for either preventative or curative treatment. Best results are achieved if the Patient prepares themselves first by being clear about what it is they need to do, and being sure they have all they need to be make themself comfortable. The process is simple, and is always easier the second time!

- Drizzle the castor oil over the cloth, not too much is required.
- Lay the cloth over the abdomen.
- Wrap cling film around the body to cover and to secure the cloth in place.
- Place a hot water bottle over the abdomen and leave for one and a half hours.

The Patient can use the time to rest, read, enjoy their favourite music, meditate, watch television, or sleep.

Of course there are many more programmes out there to choose from that once the Patient becomes familiar with their chosen approach they will find it easier to use as part of their own healthcare routines.

Diet and Nutrition

A healthy body cannot function effectively on junk food. Hence good nutrition is fundamental if good physical health is to be maintained and/or achieved. Good health cannot be taken for granted and we have to take personal responsibility for it. Disease rarely happens by accident!

A skilled colon hydrotherapist will also use dietary change as a primary source of treatment.

Nutrition is both the process by which we take in and utilize food, and the study of diet **as it relates to health. Food is converted to energy** which is used to keep us, the organism, alive. This energy is supplied by the process of **combustion or oxidation** of appropriate foodstuffs in the tissues which also results in the production of heat. The continuous work of the tissues means that wear and tear will take place requiring repair. Materials are needed for this purpose and for growth. **Our food must therefore address three purposes:**

- The provision of energy and heat (carbohydrates and fats)
- The requirement for body-building and repair (proteins)
- The regulating of vital processes (vitamins and minerals)

The series of changes involving the building up and breaking down of food substances is called **metabolism**. The chemical changes involved in the breaking down of worn-out tissues, and their removal, is called **katabolism.** The building up of fresh tissues from nutritive materials supplied in the food is called **anabolism.** In health there is a balance between anabolism and katabolism.

For such chemical changes to occur, the changes involve the consumption of a large amount of oxygen which must be absorbed into the bloodstream and conveyed to the tissues where the chemical changes take place. Nutritional energy, **calories,** originates in solar energy and is absorbed by foods through photosynthesis. (A calorie is defined as the amount of heat required to raise 1l (1000ml) of water 1°C).

The requirements of a healthy diet are:

- To contain sufficient **calorific value** (a moderately active women aged 18 to 55 would eat around 1,800 calories a day with around 1,080 from carbohydrate. Her male counterpart, needing about 2,300 calories a day should get up to 1,380 carbohydrate calories per day. (Weil A, 2002)

- To contain **protein** (20%, there is concern that we consume too much protein, the quality of the protein is as important as the quantity). **Fat and oils** (30%, with 5% of calories from saturated fat, 20% of calories from monounsaturated fat (best sources, olive oil, canola oil), and the remaining 5% from polyunsaturated fat). **Carbohydrate** (50%, from low GI and high-fibre foods). These proportions are a useful guide.

- To contain **fresh foods**, green vegetables and fruit in order to provide, vitamins, and fibre/roughage to stimulate the action of the bowel.

- To contain a proportion of **minerals** especially those of sodium, calcium, potassium, and iron.

- To contain an adequate amount of **water.**

- To also be palatable, visually appetizing, and **easily digested.**

In discussing nutrition it is best to separate nutrients into their various parts. These consist of: **proteins, carbohydrates, fats and oils, vitamins, minerals, and dietary fibre.**

The most important matter is of course the quality of the food we eat!

Protein

The word **protein** means, 'of primary importance', and proteins are complex compounds containing nitrogen, sulphur, phosphorous, carbon, hydrogen, and oxygen. These enter into the composition of protoplasm itself. (Remember: the smallest living unit of the body is the cell which is a mass of protoplasm containing a nucleus). Protein is broken down into digestive ferments and absorbed into the blood.

There are two types of protein: **animal protein,** (includes myosin, albumen, globulin) found in meats, fish, cheese and eggs, and **vegetable protein,** (includes gluten, legumin) found in wheat, beans, and lentils (the leguminous plants, legumes are dried beans).

189

Protein is our building food and our major source of heat energy. It can be converted into fat and stored in the body. Proteins are broken down by the digestive process into their basic constituents which are **amino acids.** These amino acids are then absorbed and synthesized into more protein and **enzymes** and constituents that the body needs.

Enzymes are catalysts for digestion and metabolism of food. They are destroyed at 41.5°C (107°F). They are secreted by the alimentary canal glands and some are in the fresh food we eat. (See Table 6, Digestive Enzymes)

Different enzymes act upon particular foods: ptyalin converts starch to maltose; pepsin, proteins into peptones; rennin, milk into casein; trypsin, peptones into amino acids; amylase, all starch (cooked or uncooked) into maltose; lipase, fats into glucose; erepsin, peptones into amino acids.

Digestive enzyme supplements are available and can often assist proper digestion.

Amino acids, as noted, are the basic constituents of protein, number around 22, and all must be present in our body at the same time and in the right quantity for protein synthesis to occur. The body can manufacture all but 10 of these, the others, the **essential amino acids** must be obtained from protein within our diet.

Animal protein is always complete and will provide B12. The disadvantages include high fat and cholesterol, pollutants, lack of fibre, and sometimes poor treatment of the animals. Vegetable and fruits are incomplete proteins and are low in one or more of the essential amino acids. Vegetable source protein must be combined if it is to be a reliable source of the essential amino acids.

A diet of mainly combined vegetable source protein (including grains/legumes) with small amounts of animal source protein, for example, a vegetarian who eats some dairy and eggs and a small amount of fish seems to work well for many people.

Remember, excessive consumption of animal protein leads to an acid constitution, with excess ureas in the tissues which is the primary cause of many degenerative diseases, especially inflammatory conditions such as arthritis. Protein deficiency will result in low energy and stamina, poor resistance to infection, slow healing of wounds, and prolonged recovery from illness.

Requiring special comment is the fact, as noted above, that vegetable protein lacks the vitamin B12 (found only in foods of animal origin). B12 combines with the intrinsic factor and prevents pernicious anaemia. B12 is essential for the development of red blood cells in the bone marrow. The body can store this vitamin and needs only miniscule amounts of it each day. Unless their diet includes some fish, eggs, or dairy products people should take B12 in the form of a supplement.

The traditional view was that we require around 70g of protein a day. Current research has concluded that large amounts of protein are not necessarily required, and indeed may be quite damaging. Around 20 to 30g per day is now suggested. Much of this evidence also suggests that combined vegetable proteins are of a superior quality to animal protein. (School of Natural Health Sciences, 2007). (To convert grams to ounces multiply by 0.0352, meaning that 3g s equivalent to just over 1 ounce).

Vegans and vegetarians are frequently questioned about their respective sources of protein. Although protein is an essential nutrient which plays many important roles in the way the body functions it is not difficult to get the recommended daily allowance of around 0.8 grams of protein for every kilogram that we weigh (or about 0.36g of protein for pound that we weigh). (Food and Nutrition Board, Institute of Medicine, 2002). (See Table 8. The Protein Content of Selected Vegan Foods).

Carbohydrates

Carbohydrates are the most readily available source of energy and consist of carbon, hydrogen, and oxygen, but in a totally different chemical combination to that of fat. Carbohydrates are widely distributed throughout the animal and vegetable kingdoms but are especially found in the latter. They include starches, sugar, and cellulose and are present in grains, fruits, and vegetables.

Carbohydrates are easily digested and broken down by enzyme action into glucose, in which form they are absorbed, producing heat and energy. Any excess is converted into fat and stored in the tissues.

The refining of carbohydrates strips them of their fibre, and the loss of nearly all their B vitamins, vitamin E, and minerals. They become indigestible, valueless, and constipating and cause problems with the body's sugar economy, for example, **hypoglycaemia** and possibly diabetes. A large amount of carbohydrates, eaten daily, requires the pancreas to work harder. This is because **insulin** is required to manage the flood of glucose into the bloodstream, which follows every high-carbohydrate meal. Symptoms include: erratic mood swings, sugar cravings and energy lows, irritability and depression, trembling and palpitations, menstrual problems, and hormonal disturbance.

Sugar consumption is very much linked to the stress in life and vice versa. The result is a continuous strain on the pancreas and as a result it begins to over-respond by producing too much insulin, thus too much sugar is broken down and the Patient ends up with not enough in the blood stream. The consequence is hypoglycaemia.

The GI is the measure of how different carbohydrate foods affect blood glucose. The higher the GI level, the faster is the rate of increase of glucose in the blood, the greater the insulin response, and the greater the potential to expose the body to the toxic effects of high blood sugar, and harmful effects of insulin, for example, encouraging the body to store up calories as fat, can promote arterial damage, and may accelerate the growth of tumours.

Foods with GI levels below 55 are considered to have a low GI. Numbers above 70 indicate a high GI, and numbers between 55 and

70 are intermediate. Because of refinement processes, sugar and salt additives and poor production many of us will be consuming carbohydrates from high GI foods and carbohydrates of poor quality.

The issue is to ensure the majority of carbohydrate calories come from low GI whole-grains, beans, and vegetables; and low GI fruits like berries, apples, and cherries. It is also possible to reduce the impact of higher GI foods by eating them as part of mixed meals including fibre and acid (lemon and vinegar) and eating them in moderation and with low GI foods at the same meal.

Fats and Oils

Fats and Oils (or lipids – fats, oils, fatty acids, and compounds derived from them) are the most concentrated source of energy in our diet. They are used as a source of energy, and as building and repair molecules and they provide the fat soluble vitamins A D E F and K. One gram of fat will yield nine calories of energy to the body.

Essential fatty acids (for example, omega-3, sources include fish oil and linseed oil, and omega-6, sources include evening primrose oil and egg yolk) are the building blocks of fat. Some can be synthesized by the body, others, the essential fatty acids, must be obtained from the diet.

Saturated fats and oils (sources include animal fat, butter fat, coconut oil, palm oil), show that those from animal sources, are usually hard at room temperature. **Mono-unsaturated fats** (sources include avocado oil, olive oil, almond oil, sesame oil, canola oil, hazelnut oil) and **polyunsaturated fats** (sources include fish oil, linseed oil, soybean oil, walnut oil, and sunflower oil) come mainly from vegetables, nut, and seed sources are usually liquid at room temperature.

Eating too many saturated fats is the major cause of coronary heart disease, and in most cases they contain large amounts of cholesterol. Saturated fats block the arteries and slow down the removal of waste matter and toxins by clogging the lymphatic system.

193

Monounsaturated and polyunsaturated fats will help prevent heart disease by preventing the build-up of fatty deposits and should be in their natural form only. When they are hardened or hydrogenated (combined with hydrogen, for the making of such processed foods as margarine, low-fat spreads), their chemical structure changes and they behave in the body like saturated fats.

Polyunsaturated fats contain essential fatty acids which are absolutely essential for life. (omega-6 comes from linoleic acid found in most vegetable oils and nuts and omega-3 found mainly in fish oils). The body can make its own supply of mono-unsaturates; polyunsaturates must come from the food we eat. Only small amounts are required daily.

All fats and oils are mixtures of fatty acids. Fat and carbohydrates are clean-burning fuels releasing only carbon dioxide and water as the final by-products of **oxidation.** Protein, in addition, leaves a residue of ammonia, a compound of nitrogen and hydrogen. This is extremely toxic, especially to brain cells, and therefore excess consumption of protein may increase the workload on the liver and kidneys regarding elimination.

Remember, the enzyme lipase converts/splits fats into fatty acids and glycerine. For the purpose of absorption of digested fats the presence of **bile salts** is necessary. Fatty acids and glycerine are absorbed into the villi of the small intestine and are recombined to form saturated fats. These, unlike glucose and aminoacids, enter the lacteals of the villi and not the bloodstream directly.

From the lacteals of the villi they pass via the cisterna chyli and thoracic duct (lymphatic vessels) to the bloodstream which takes them to fat stores of the body. When they are required, they are conveyed to the liver and then tissues where they are converted into carbon dioxide and water, with the production of heat. (See The Five Systems of Elimination section).

Oxidants are molecules derived from normal intracellular processes and released by inflammatory cells. They **are unstable and**

194

dangerous because they have an uneven electrical charge. Oxidative stress upon the body occurs when **oxygen reacts with fats/oils** causing the formation of a range of dangerous compounds called **free radicals.**

Such free radicals with unpaired electrons are unstable and have a high oxidation potential, which means they are capable of stealing electrons from other cells. This chemical mechanism is useful in disinfectants, such as hydrogen peroxide and ozone, which can be used to sterilise wounds or medical instruments. Inside the body these free radicals are also of great benefit due to their ability to attack and eliminate bacteria, viruses, and other waste products.

However, problems arise when too many of these free radicals are turned loose in the body where they can damage normal tissue and an array of unpleasant substances are created, such as: **hydrogen sulphide, ammonia, histamines, indoles, phenols, and scatoles.** (These substances are also produced naturally in the digestive tract when we digest food, resulting in the unpleasant odour evidenced in faeces).

Putrefaction of spoiled food is caused by microbes in the air. This natural process is duplicated in the digestive tract by intestinal microbes. All these waste products are pathogenic, thus able to cause disease in the body.

Hydrogen sulphide and ammonia are tissue toxins that can damage the liver. Histamines contribute to allergic disorders such as: atopic dermatitis, urticaria (hives), and asthma. (Patients with a predisposition to react to given allergens are described as atopic). Indoles and phenols are considered to be carcinogenic.

Free radicals are also be caused by environmental factors, for example, perfumes, paint, exhaust fumes, cigarettes, food additives, alcohol, and drugs. The body must defend against free radicals by relying upon **antioxidants.** Antioxidants can block the damage. These are compounds which quench free radicals and neutralise the destructive oxidation reactions, for example, premature ageing, heart disease, cancer, and allergies. **The best- known sources of antioxidants are whole foods.**

Cholesterol is a lipid and is often supplied with saturated fats and oils. It is part of all cell membranes, and is a major component of brain tissue, nerve tissue, the liver, and the blood. It is the precursor of steroid hormones (mainly adrenal and sex hormones) and is needed for vitamin D synthesis and the production of bile from the liver. Clearly, cholesterol is vitally important to the functioning of the body, however, most of the cholesterol that we need is manufactured by the liver (85%).

We only require a small amount from dietary sources. Excessive dietary cholesterol will contribute, as noted above, to blocking of the arteries and blood vessels, and may lead to fatal disorders.

A common medical diagnostic test is the **'serum lipid profile'** to measure levels of fat and cholesterol in the body. High levels usually result from overeating, especially the eating of refined carbohydrate with a high GI.

It is recommended to reduce the amount of saturated fat in the diet, or try low-fat forms. Avoid heating any oil to the point of smoking and never breathe smoke of heated or burning fat as it is highly toxic. Avoid fried food and margarine. Use extra virgin olive oil as your main fat.

Vitamins and Minerals

Vitamins are organic nutrients (meaning they contain the element carbon) and are required by the body in minute quantities in order to maintain growth and normal metabolism. Minerals are inorganic substances and are the most permanent part of living things. They do not burn, and can in fact be found in the ashes of something that has burned.

Unlike proteins, fats, or carbohydrates, vitamins do not provide energy or serve as building materials. Their function is the

regulation of physical processes. Most serve as **co-enzymes,** (supporting the reaction which is catalysed by the given enzyme). Avitaminosis refers to a deficiency of any vitamin. Hyper-vitaminosis refers to an excess of one or more vitamins.

There are **two major groups** of vitamins: These are:

- Water-soluble vitamins: B, C, and P, the bioflavinoids, and these assist in the absorption of vitamin C and increasing the strength and permeability of the capillaries, called the P factor. Bioflavinoids always accompany vitamin C in nature. These are not stored for long in our bodies, around three days only, therefore we require a regular supply.

- Fat-soluble vitamins A D E F and K, are stored in the body but caution must be observed with supplemental fat soluble vitamins because excess build-up can be harmful.

Vitamin deficiency may arise from: inadequate diet, impaired absorption, insufficient utilisation, and increased excretion. Deficiency develops in two stages: sub-clinical deficiency, the depletion of the body's stores, and overt deficiency is usually evidence of malnutrition. (See Table 2: Vitamins).

Minerals are mostly inorganic substances. They make up about 5% of our bodyweight and are found mostly in the skeleton. **Minerals and trace minerals** are absolutely essential for life and the deficiency of a mineral can be very serious.

There are 28 naturally occurring essential elements. People whose diets are deficient in particular vitamins or minerals will benefit from **supplementation**. For example, persons with adult-onset diabetes are often deficient in chromium and may have better sugar levels if they take that mineral in supplemental form.

However, taking more of these minerals, if they are not required, is not going to improve the Patient's health and may have harmful effects. For example, supplemental iron can be dangerously toxic if not needed. Be cautious of iron supplements, check first through blood tests via the Patient's Doctor that a deficiency exists.

197

It is very important to understand that mega-dose supplementation **is a therapeutic process.** Therapeutic processes, whether dietary, vitamin, or mineral supplements, are about correcting deficiencies and supporting healing and renewed balance. An oversupply can create an imbalance of other nutrients. For example, long-term use of zinc will block iron and copper absorption; too much sodium may contribute to high blood pressure.

The prescribing of supplements is often part of the colon hydrotherapy treatment plan. Such will need to be monitored very carefully in the knowledge that intolerances can also develop, when used repeatedly, to supplement use just as they can with foods. Supplementation is one part of the therapeutic process and is therefore monitored accordingly.

Remember that restrictive diets or large doses of nutrients/ supplements may be appropriate for two weeks, one month, or even three months. However, doses for periods longer than this may risk an oversupply. As we have already recognized, many Patients require supplements because of nutritional shortfalls. The more such problems are overcome, the less will be the need for supplements. As part of an ongoing treatment plan and supplement use, the application of maintenance doses only, is recommended.

The **essential major minerals** include calcium, magnesium, phosphorous, sodium, chlorine, sulphur, potassium, iron, manganese, and zinc. **Essential trace minerals** include copper, selenium, and chromium. The **ultra-trace minerals** include arsenic, boron, cadmium, lead, nickel, tin, bromium, silicon, and vanadium. (See Table 3: Minerals, Introduction and Summary Tables).

In addition to the above elements, our body requires hydrogen, nitrogen, oxygen, and carbon. These are available in either the air we breathe or as components of all the living matter we eat.

Major minerals are needed in the diet in amounts of 100mg or more per day. As you know a milligram is a very small amount, being one-thousandth of a gram, and there are 28g in an ounce. Trace minerals are needed in smaller amounts, less than 100mg per day. The ultra-trace minerals are required in quantities of less than 1mg per day, and are toxic in larger doses, and remember excess of any mineral can be dangerous.

Minerals by themselves are inactive chemical elements, but in the body they are used in many different ways. For example, iron is used to carry oxygen to the cells; calcium is used to make bones and teeth; sodium, potassium, and chloride are called 'electrolytes' and they maintain water balance and provide the correct pressure between cells and their surrounding fluids.

Many minerals need to 'partner up' with an amino acid before they can be accepted onto a receptor sight on the intestine wall. Hence the term 'chelated' mineral. Chelated means 'bind to' and supplemental chelated minerals are those which have been chemically bound to a suitable amino acid. This removes their requirement to do it in the gut and therefore greatly improves the absorptive ability of the mineral supplement. Examples would be calcium chelate, or magnesium chelate. A more specific example is calcium orotate, which is calcium bound to an amino acid, that is, orotic acid. Orotates are highly absorbable in bone.

In the body, minerals:

- Become part of tissue structure.
- Help maintain acid-base balance and keep the body pH neutral.
- Regulate body processes such as enzyme systems.
- Function in nerve impulse transmission and muscle contraction.
- Help in the release of energy from food.

Minerals are present in all foods but in different amounts, and all foods do not contain the same minerals. This is why we need to eat a variety of good quality and nutritious foods.

Dietary Fibre

Dietary fibre, or roughage, is the **indigestible part of food** that makes up much of the bulk of stool. Adequate peristalsis in the bowel only occurs when there is sufficient fibre for the muscle in the colon wall to act upon. This is because the normal **stimulus to peristaltic action** is the stretching of the walls by the degree of content actually contained within the bowel.

Dietary fibre is a generic term. It includes the following **chemicals** which form the structural components of plants, including many of the plant foods we eat: cellulose, hemicelluloses, lignin, pectins, mucilages, and gums. The first three are insoluble fibres which can absorb and hold water in the digestive system. The others are soluble fibres which are partly broken down in digestion to a gel-like substance, which also retains water.

By ensuring fibre in the diet **intestinal disorders** will be **minimized.** Fibre in foods like berries and other fresh fruits, vegetables, whole grains, seeds, and nuts is known to reduce the risk of obesity, diabetes, high blood cholesterol, cardiovascular disease, and numerous gastrointestinal disorders, for example: constipation, inflammatory bowel disease, colitis, haemorrhoids, Crohn's disease, diverticulitis, and colon cancer.

Low-fibre faeces are dehydrated and hardened, thus making them difficult to evacuate. Dietary fibre includes non-starch polysaccharides (NSP) and oligosaccharides that cannot be digested in the small intestine by alpha-amylase or any of the sugar hydrolysing enzymes in the gut.

Fibre is characterized as soluble or insoluble.

Soluble fibre sources include: legumes, (peas, soybeans, and other beans). Fruits and fruit juices (especially prune juice, plums, apples, and berries). Vegetables, especially leafy green varieties, and oats. Root vegetables such as potatoes, sweet potatoes, and onions and the *psyllium* seed husk (often used as a bulk-forming laxative).

Insoluble fibre sources include: wholegrain foods, bran, nuts, and seeds, vegetables such as green beans, cauliflower, celery, and the skins of some fruits.

Soluble dietary fibre, as well as lowering blood cholesterol, is also involved in the regulation of blood-sugar levels. Insoluble dietary fibre is essential in assisting in maintaining optimal bowel movements. Dietary fibre contains no calories. Animal products contain no fibre unless the formulated product has dietary fibre added. (See Table 4, Fibre Content of Some Foods).

The values in Table 4 are reported as grams per hundred grams of edible portion. (100g equals 3.5 ounces). Information is given in the conversion column so that the value can be converted to the foods normally eaten.

The cooking itself does not generally alter the fibre content of foods unless the water content is changed in the process. The cooking of vegetables will break down the cell-wall structure and therefore soften tissues. However, this does not remove the polysaccharides associated with the cell wall.

The ability of fibre to hold water, to bind to minerals and cholesterol-like materials, results in **a number of physiological effects.** These effects vary depending on the type of fibre, and/or where it is in the digestive tract. For example:

- In the mouth, fibre helps stimulate the flow of saliva.

- In the stomach and small intestine, fibre dilutes the contents and delays the emptying of food and the absorption of nutrients (this promotes a feeling of fullness).

- In the large intestine, fibre also acts to bind certain chemicals. Different kinds of fibre have different binding capacities as when fibre binds cholesterol-like compounds it lowers cholesterol. Fibre does not bind to minerals and vitamins and therefore does not restrict their absorption, but rather, evidence exists that fer-mentable fibre sources improve absorption of minerals, especially calcium. (ncbi.nlm.nih.gov).

The net effect of all the points discussed is that a diet high in fibre-rich foods is likely to cause digestion and absorption to occur along a greater length of the small intestines. Because fibre is not digested it passes into the bowel where it can remain undigested and serve as a substrate for the micro-flora normally present.

Fibre is the only dietary component that causes stool weight and fibre has specific attributes that promote the normal functioning of the gastrointestinal tract, including defecation. Because fibre is a resistant carbohydrate, eating more of it may cause flatulence and bloating for the same reason that beans are gas producing. Bacteria in the gut attack and digest the complex carbohydrate, releasing methane gas in the process.

A healthy adult requires 20–25g of fibre a day (based on the assumption that we need 10–13g of fibre for every 1,000 calories consumed). Many people consume only about 10g of fibre each day.

Remember, two or more dessertspoons of linseeds, soaked in water if preferred, and consumed in the morning; is a bulking fibre; is high in essential fatty acids and linolenic acid (omega-3), which is the biochemical precursor to body's anti-inflammatory prostaglandi ns. (Therefore it helps to calm IBS and colitis). Psyllium husks produce a soft, cooling lubricant which absorbs poisons and reduces inflammation. Slippery elm protects the intestinal walls from toxins and acids.

Acid and Alkaline Balance:

The acid and alkaline balance within the body, the **pH level,** is the acid and alkaline measurement of internal fluids, and this balance has an enormous impact on a person's health.

When the body is acidic it begins to retain water to buffer the acidity; retains fat to bind acid and take it away from internal organs; creates cholesterol to protect the cells of the arterial walls from acid damage; leeches minerals from bones and tissues in its attempt to neutralize acidity and

this can lead to the formation of stones, osteoporosis, or muscle breakdown; forms tumours to encapsulate morbid cells and their associated acids, all these processes indicate a body in 'self-preservation' mode!

Every cell in the body is affected, and when the pH gets out of balance (for example, too acidic) the Patient may experience low energy, fatigue, excess weight, poor digestion, aches and pains, and even more serious disorders. Chronic acidity (acidosis) will interrupt all cellular activity and functions, interfering with life itself!

Moreover, as we age we lose bicarbonate in our blood which is an alkaline buffer that neutralizes acid. Therefore, lack of bicarbonate causes an accumulation of acid in the body which is a primary cause of poor blood circulation and degenerative diseases.

Virtually all **degenerative diseases** including cancer, heart disease, arthritis, osteoporosis, kidney and gall stones, and tooth decay, are associated with excess acidity in the body. **We need to understand the simple process of alkalizing the body and the important role a properly alkalized body plays in restoring and maintaining overall health.** Our glands and organs function, in exact proportion to, the alkaline and acid levels with in our system.

Bicarbonate is a major element of the body. Bicarbonate compounds include: sodium, potassium, and calcium. Secreted by the stomach it is necessary for digestion and is present in all body fluids. The stomach has 30 million glands that produce gastric juice containing not only acids but also bicarbonate, which reduces the acidity of dietary compounds such as protein.

When acidity of the body reduces so will the excess weight of the body. How we feel and think will also be affected. Therefore, obesity is not a fat problem but an excess acid problem and the body's inability to remove its own dietary waste products. Paradoxically, the retention of fat helps to maintain the pH level of the blood as a result of the body being too acidic!

'The digestive system is not designed for the digestion of

food but designed for the alkalizing of food in preparation for becoming blood and then new body cells'. (Young R, Omaha Lecture 2007, YouTube).

Therefore, diet influences acid-alkaline balance both through the acid or alkaline-forming nature of the foods that are eaten as well as through the nutrient content which affects metabolism. We can remain healthy by consuming a diet that is 70 to 80% alkaline and 20 to 30% acid. Most raw foods are predominantly alkaline-forming foods. (See Table 7, Food Types and pH Levels). Alkalinity is anabolic (building) whereas acidity is catabolic (breaking down).

An acid is a substance that increases the concentration of hydrogen ions (H+) in water. On the pH scale, which ranges from 0 at the acid end to 14 on the alkaline end, a solution is neutral if its pH is 7. At pH 7, water contains equal concentrations of H+ and OH- ions. Substances with a pH less than 7 are acidic. **Substances higher than 7 are alkaline.**

The pH scale is a logarithm scale so a change of 1pH unit means a ten-fold change in the concentration of hydrogen ions. In other words, a ph of 5 is 10 times more acid than 6, 100 times more acid than 7 and 1,000 times more acid than 8. Given this information it is easy to see how a slight change in pH value can have a major impact on our internal environment.

Living things are extremely sensitive to pH changes and function best when solutions are nearly neutral. Exceptions, for example, include parts of the digestive tract; and further examples evidence that crabs die at acid pH6; fish and all living marine life die at pH3; a can of soft drink often has a pH2.5 which is highly acid.

Optimum alkalinity at the cellular level equates to optimum health. We live and die at the cellular level. **A healthy person's pH level** of their body fluids should be between 7.1 and 7.5. The 75 trillion cells of the body, in health, are alkaline. In disease, the cell pH is below 7. The more acid the cell becomes the sicker the Patient will be. A range from 6.5 is weakly acidic to 4.5 which is strongly acidic. Most children have a

7.5 pH. Over half of adults have pH6.5 or lower (reflecting calcium deficiency and effects of lifestyle). (Baroody T A, 2005). It is the potassium, calcium, and sodium minerals which neutralise the unhealthy toxic waste. These minerals are found in alkaline-forming foods.

Blood plasma and other fluids that surround cells in the body have a pH of 7.36 to 7.42. The saliva pH in a healthy person is 7.1 to 7.5.

The pH of the spinal fluid is 7.4. Lymph fluids and the fluids that are inside or that surround cells prefer the 7.39 measurement. The body's pancreatic juices have a pH range between 7.5 and 8.8. The pH of urine can go as high as 6 or as low as 4.5. The reason that urine can tolerate such a range is because urine does not stay inside the body very long. It is regularly eliminated. The outer layers of the skin have a pH of 5.2 thus enabling the skin to meet one of its primary functions which is to kill microbes so they are unable to enter the body. The inner layers of the skin have a ph of 7.35. (Vasey C, 2005).

In health, the pH of the stomach, urine, colon, and skin should be slightly acid. There is a significant variation between the pH levels in the stomach, small intestine, and colon. The stomach pH ranges from 1.5 to 3.0. If too little acid is produced in the stomach then its ability to break down food, and also kill harmful bacteria, will be affected. If acid production is too high the result will be ulcers.

After leaving the stomach, food enters the duodenum, pH4.0 to 5.0, then the small intestine (jejunum and ileum) which has an alkaline pH of 6.5 to 8. The colon pH is around 5.6 to 6.9, which is a slightly acid pH. (Webster D, 1999). When the colon is too alkaline the protective bacteria found naturally within the colon do not flourish. This then encourages the growth of opportunistic flora such as *candida albicans.*

As we can see parts of the body need to function at different acid and alkaline levels. What is important is to take steps to return the body's respective internal biochemical environment to its natural and proper pH level, thus, reversing the Patients' acidic system so they can begin to experience better health, more energy, and more vitality, with pH levels corresponding to the exact needs of the body. Remember, the natural ratio between acid and alkaline foods in the diet should be **four parts alkaline to one part acid.**

The characteristics of a diet which summarises the body's needs will:

- Avoid the intake of any harmful elements.

- Accommodate all the nutritional elements necessary to support health.

- Contain a predominance of fresh foods.

- Contain primarily unprocessed foods.

- Include an abundance of fresh fruits and vegetable.

- Eat as much raw food as possible.

- Show variety so that eating is a source of pleasure.

Therefore, a diet which reflects the above characteristics will provide for:

- An acid/alkaline balance, and adequate fibre to increase bulk for better elimination and detoxification.

- Feeding friendly bacteria and lowering cholesterol.

- Contains essential fatty acids for bowel lubrication, support of the nervous system, and stimulation of bile production for detoxification.

- Provides for hormonal, metabolic, and immune system support.

- Provides for a sustainable source of energy, is alkaline and will therefore further support detoxification, help dissolve calcium build-up, and neutralise acid from metabolism.

- Provide for a reliable source of minerals.

Summary and Conclusion

Never neglect giving attention to the colon and never, given the caveats discussed, hesitate to have colon hydrotherapy. Every part of the body will benefit. To maintain a clean colon is the best health insurance policy one can obtain. The colon provides a true insight, an indicator, of a Patient's habits and the condition of their body, whether healthy or not.

Prevention and health education is always close to the heart of a colon hydrotherapist. Moreover, the committed and skilled Practitioner will always be active regarding their continuous professional development, ongoing study, improving their knowledge, professional abilities, and exploring ways in which new skills can be utilized in their own practice so that outcomes for the Patient may be enhanced.

Few of us reach perfection. There will always be matters to work through and ways in which to improve. The process of change for all of us can sometimes be frightening and worrying. Such new strains or goals need to be handled, endured, and coped with in the process of personal growth and the target of achieving and maintaining optimum health. With support, guidance, and empowerment, each of us can, if we so choose, take responsibility for functioning differently and achieving new life goals.

Figure 1: The Colon

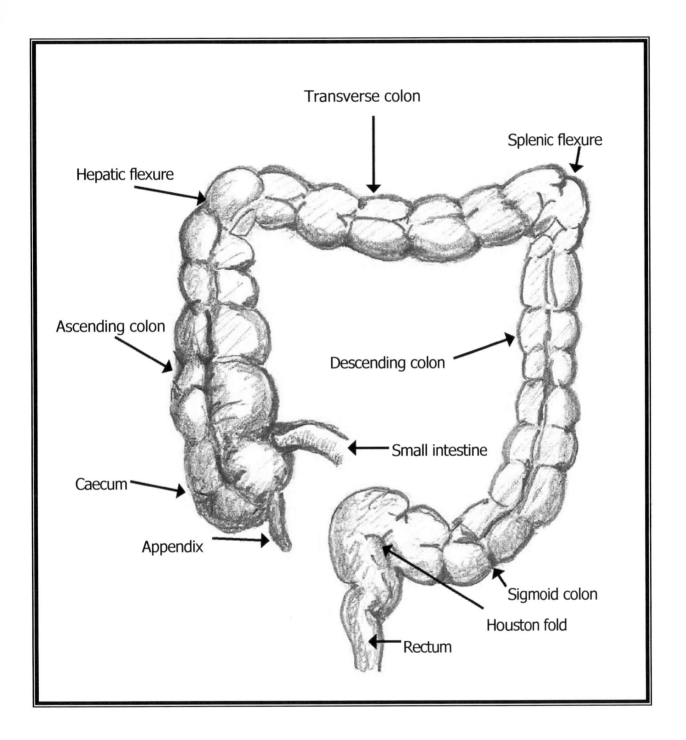

Figure 2: Food Transit Times

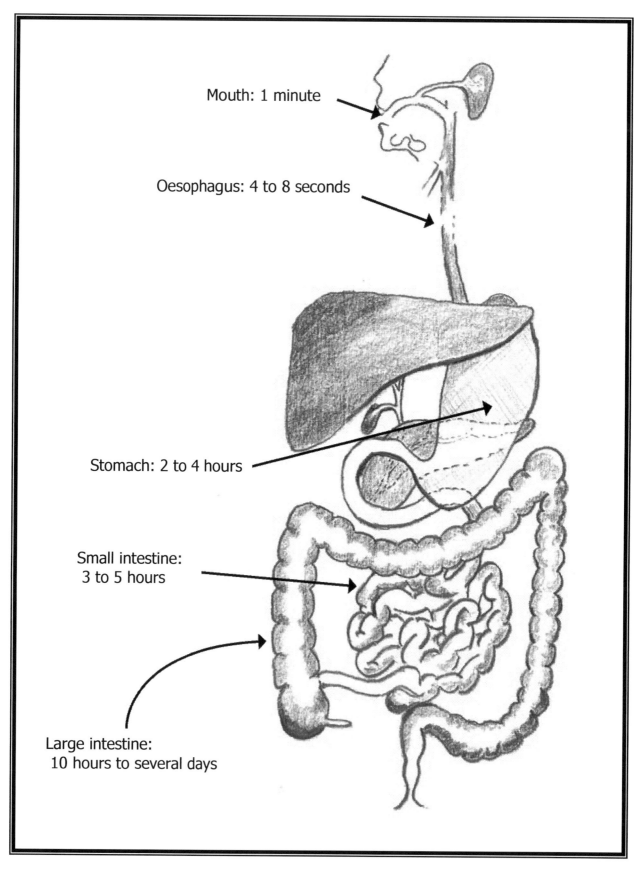

Mouth: 1 minute

Oesophagus: 4 to 8 seconds

Stomach: 2 to 4 hours

Small intestine:
3 to 5 hours

Large intestine:
10 hours to several days

Figure 3: Reflex Points of the Colon and their Interrelation with Anatomical Centres and Pathology (Walker N, 1979)

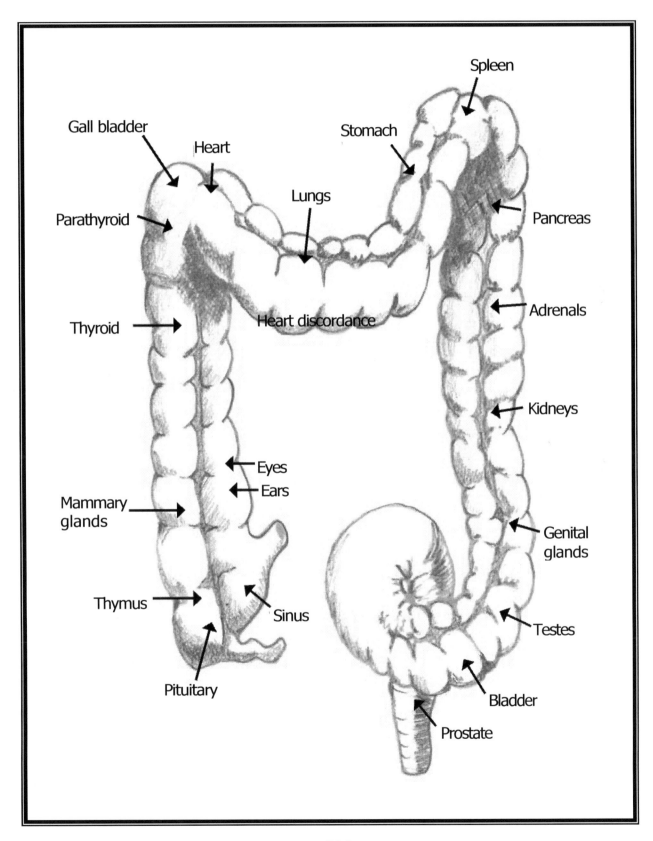

Figure 4: The Colon: Mass Peristalsis

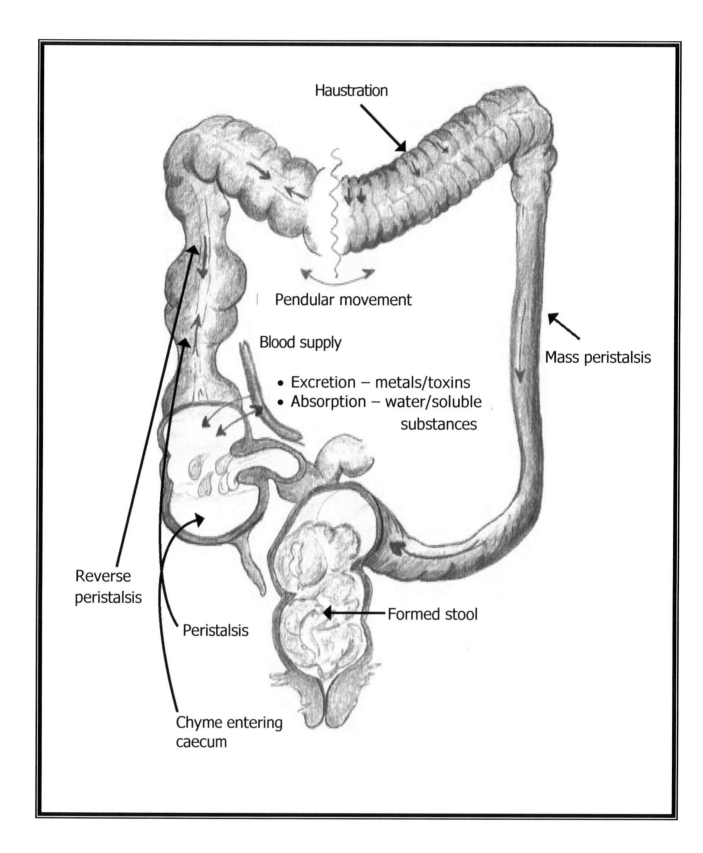

Figure 5: The Main Diseases/Conditions of the GI Tract

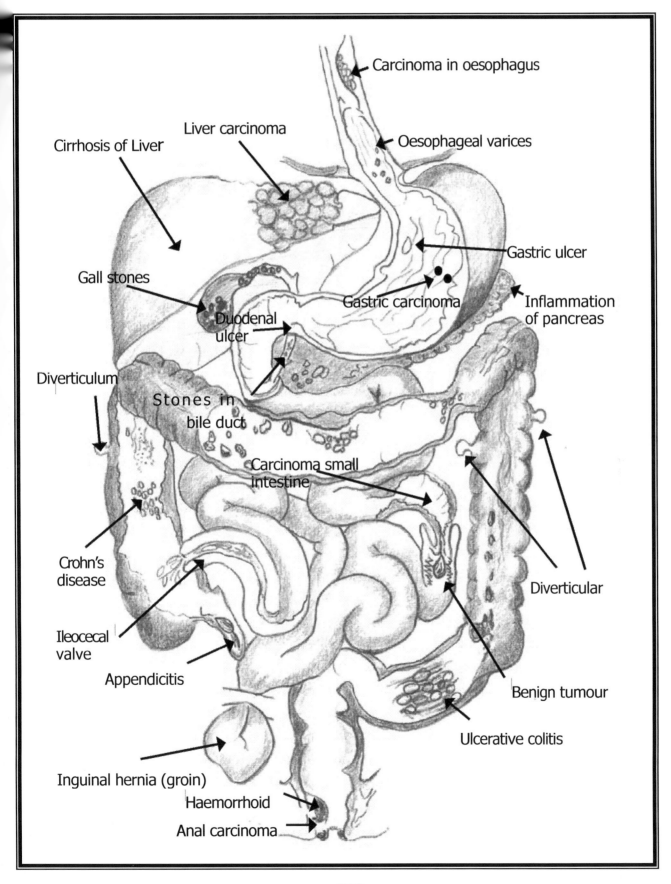

Carcinoma in oesophagus

Liver carcinoma

Oesophageal varices

Cirrhosis of Liver

Gastric ulcer

Gall stones

Gastric carcinoma

Inflammation of pancreas

Duodenal ulcer

Diverticulum

Stones in bile duct

Carcinoma small intestine

Crohn's disease

Diverticular

Ileocecal valve

Appendicitis

Benign tumour

Ulcerative colitis

Inguinal hernia (groin)

Haemorrhoid

Anal carcinoma

Figure 6: Gastrointestinal Tract

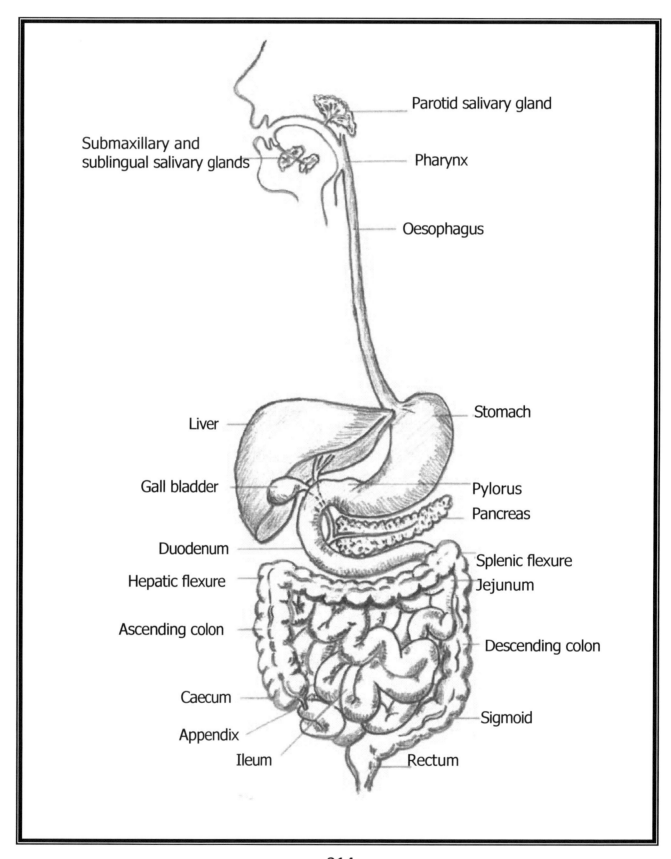

Figure 7: Pressure Points

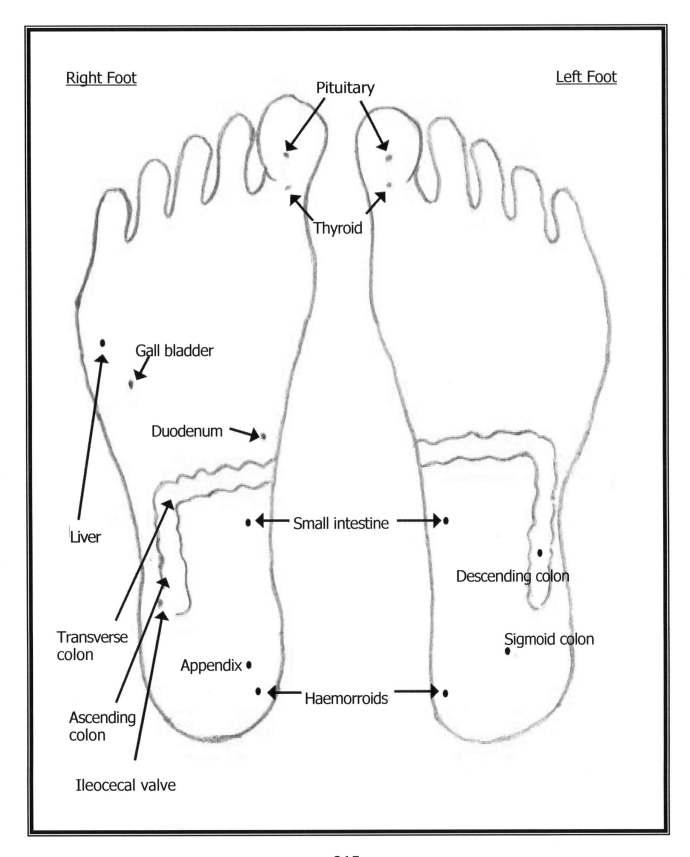

Right Foot

Left Foot

Pituitary

Thyroid

Gall bladder

Duodenum

Liver

Small intestine

Descending colon

Transverse
colon

Sigmoid colon

Appendix

Ascending
colon

Haemorroids

Ileocecal valve

Figure 7a: Pressure Points (continued)

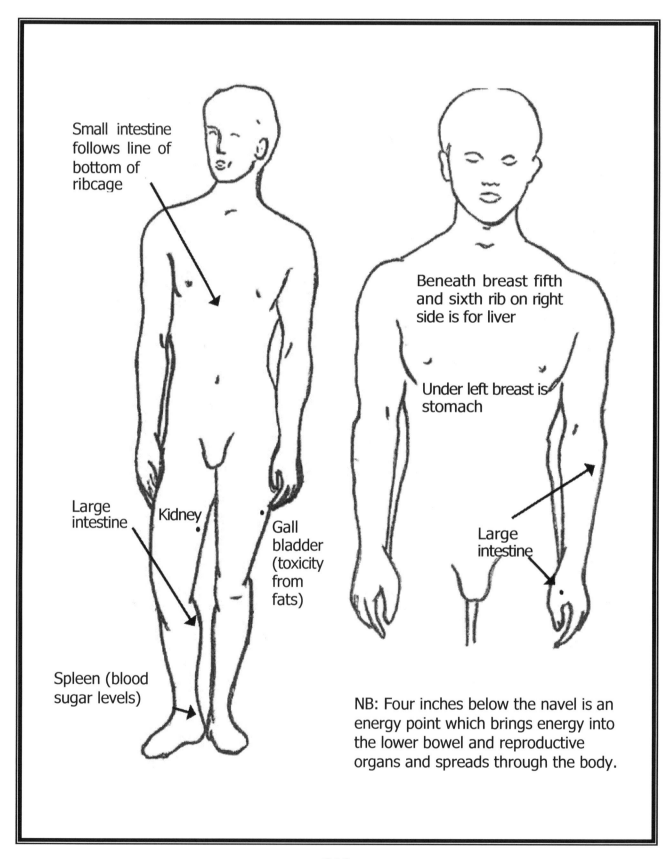

Small intestine follows line of bottom of ribcage

Large intestine

Kidney

Gall bladder (toxicity from fats)

Spleen (blood sugar levels)

Beneath breast fifth and sixth rib on right side is for liver

Under left breast is stomach

Large intestine

NB: Four inches below the navel is an energy point which brings energy into the lower bowel and reproductive organs and spreads through the body.

Table 1: Low glycemic index (GI) food (less than 55), foods with GI index between 55 and 70 are considered intermediate, high glycemic index food (more than 70)

Notes: *high in empty calories **low-calorie and nutritious foods						
Food List	**Rating**	**Food Glycem/ Index**		**Food List**	**Rating**	**Food Glycem/ Index**
Bakery Products				**Root Crop**		
*Pound cake	Low	54		Carrots, cooked	Low	39
Danish pastry	Medium	59		Yam	Low	51
Muffin (un-sweetened)	Medium	62		Sweet potato	Low	54
Cake, tart	Medium	65		Potato, boiled	Medium	56
Cake, angel	Medium	67		Potato, new	Medium	57
Croissant	Medium	67		Potato, tinned	Medium	61
Waffles	High	76		Beetroot	Medium	64
Doughnut	High	76		Potato, steamed	Medium	65
Beverages				Mashed	Medium	70
Soya milk	Low	30		Chips	High	75
Apple juice	Low	41		Potato, micro-waved	High	82
Carrot juice	Low	45		Potato, instant	High	83
Pineapple juice	Low	46		**Potato, baked	High	85
Grapefruit juice	Low	48		Parsnips	High	97
Orange juice	Low	52				
Food List	**Rating**	**Food Glycem/ Index**		**Food List**	**Rating**	**Food Glycem/ Index**
Biscuits				**Snack Food and Sweets**		
Digestives	Medium	58		Peanuts	Low	15
Shortbread	Medium	64		*M&Ms (peanut)	Low	32
Water biscuits	Medium	65		*Snickers bar	Low	40
Ryvita	Medium	67		*Chocolate bar; 30g	Low	49
Wafer biscuits	High	77		Jams and marmalades	Low	49
**Rice cakes	High	77		*Crisps	Low	54
Breads				Popcorn	Medium	55
Multigrain bread	Low	48		Mars bar	Medium	64
Wholegrain	Low	50		*Table sugar (sucrose)	Medium	65
Pita bread, white	Medium	57		Corn chips	High	74
Pizza, cheese	Medium	60		Jelly beans	High	80
Hamburger bun	Medium	61		Pretzels	High	81
Rye-flour bread	Medium	64		Dates	High	103
Wholemeal	Medium	69		**Soups**		
White bread	High	71		Tomato soup, tinned	Low	38

	Rating	Food Glycem/Index		Food List	Rating	Food Glycem/Index
White rolls	High	73		Lentil soup, tinned	Low	44
Baguette	High	95		Black bean soup, tinned	Medium	64
Dairy Foods				Green pea soup, tinned	Medium	66
Yogurt low-fat (sweetened)	Low	14				
Milk, chocolate	Low	24				
Milk, whole	Low	27				
Milk, Fat-free	Low	32				
Milk, skimmed	Low	32				
Milk, semi-skimmed	Low	34				

Food List	Rating	Food Glycem/Index		Food List	Rating	Food Glycem/Index
Vegetables and Beans				**Vegetables and Beans**		
Artichoke	Low	15		Chickpeas	Low	33
Asparagus	Low	15		Haricot beans, boiled	Low	38
Broccoli	Low	15		Black-eyed beans	Low	41
Cauliflower	Low	15		Chickpeas, tinned	Low	42
Celery	Low	15		Baked beans, tinned	Low	48
Cucumber	Low	15		Kidney beans, tinned	Low	52
Eggplant	Low	15		Lentils green, tinned	Low	52
Green beans	Low	15		Broad beans	High	79
Lettuce, all	Low	15		**Pasta**		
Low-fat yogurt, artificially	Low	15		Spaghetti, protein enriched	Low	27
Peppers, all varieties	Low	15		Fettuccine	Low	32
Snow peas	Low	15		Vermicelli	Low	35
Spinach	Low	15		Spaghetti whole-wheat	Low	37
Young summer squash	Low	15		Ravioli, meat filled	Low	39
Tomatoes	Low	15		Spaghetti, white	Low	41
Courgette	Low	15		Macaroni	Low	45
Soya beans, boiled	Low	16		Spaghetti, durum wheat	Medium	55
Peas, dried	Low	22		Macaroni cheese	Medium	64
Kidney beans, boiled	Low	29		Rice pasta, brown	High	92
Lentils green, boiled	Low	29				

Food List	Rating	Food Glycem/ Index		Food List	Rating	Food Glycem/ Index
Breakfast Cereals				**Fruits**		
All-Bran	Low	42		Cherries	Low	22
Porridge, traditional	Low	49		Grapefruit	Low	25
Oat bran	Medium	55		Apricots (dried)	Low	31
Muesli	Medium	56		Apples	Low	38
Mini Wheats (wholemeal)	Medium	57		Pears	Low	38
Shredded Wheat	Medium	69		Plums	Low	39
Golden Grahams	High	71		Peaches	Low	42
Puffed wheat	High	74		Oranges	Low	44
Weetabix	High	77		Grapes	Low	46
Rice Krispies	High	82		Kiwi fruit	Low	53
Cornflakes	High	83		Bananas	Low	54
Cereal Grains				Fruit cocktail	Medium	55
Pearl barley	Low	25		Mangoes	Medium	56
Rye	Low	34		Apricots	Medium	57
Wheat kernels	Low	41		Apricots (tinned in syrup)	Medium	64
Rice, instant	Low	46		Raisins	Medium	64
Rice, par-boiled	Low	48		Pineapple	Medium	66
Barley, cracked	Low	50		**Watermelon	High	72
Rice, brown	Medium	55				
Rice, wild	Medium	57				
Rice, white	Medium	58				
Barley, flakes	Medium	66				
Taco shell	Medium	68				
Millet	High	71				

www.southbeach-diet

219

Table 2: Vitamins

Name	Main occurrence	Effectiveness	Lack of	Increased need	Characteristics	Daily need
Vitamin A (Retinol)	Cod-liver oil, liver, kidney, milk products, butter, yolk, as provitamin A in carrots	Normal growth, function and protection of skin, eyes and mucous membrane	Growth stop, night blindness	Smoker, vegetarian, in case of high alcohol consumption, intake of cathartic, birth control pill, antibiotics	Fat-soluble, light and oxygen-sensitively	approx. 1-5mg
Vitamin B1 (Thiamin)	Wheat germs, wholemeal cereals, peas, heart, pork, barm, oatmeal, liver, brown rice	Important for the nerve system, liver damage, inefficiency, pregnancy, mosquito protection (high-dosed), production of energy, affects the carbohydrates metabolism, important for the thyroid function	Heavy muscle- and nerve disturbances, tiredness, dyspepsias, dropsy, cardiac insufficiency, cramps, paralyses, prickle in arms and legs	Diet, youth, pregnant and nursing women, alcohol consumption, intake of birth control pill, antibiotics, chemotherapye	Water-soluble, Thiamin gets destroyed by heat and long storage, but not by freezing. Daily intake of vitamin B1 is important, because the body can´t store B1, which comes over the food	approx. 2mg (At carbohydrates-packed nutrition)
Vitamin B2 (Riboflavin)	Milk products, Meat, wholemeal cereal, cheese, eggs, liver, sea-fish, green leafy vegetables, whey powder	Important for body growth, untilization of fats, protein and carbohydrates, well for skin, eyes and nails, important energy bringer, oxygen transport	(Rarely) skin inflammation, brittle nails, anaemia, callus attrition	Pregnancy, intake of birth control pill and antibiotics, chemotherapy, fever, smoker, the elderly	Water-soluble, food with Vitamin B2 should be stored cool and dark.	approx. 2mg
Vitamin B3 (Niacin, Nicotine acid)	Peanuts, peas, liver, poultry, fish, lean meat	Building and degradation of fat, protein and carbohydrates, good sleep	Skin and mucosa inflammation, headache, trembling, vertigo, sleep disturbance, depressions, feeling of prickle and deafness in the limbs	Labor, fever, nursing women	Water-soluble, effect is outweighed by sugar and alcohol	13-16mg
Vitamin B5 (Pantothen acid)	Liver, vegetable, wheat germs, asparagus, crabs, meat, sunflower cores, pumpernickel	Against turning grey, hair loss, hair and mucous membrane illnesses, necessary for the dismantling of fat, proteins and carbohydrates	Nerve malfunctions, bad healing of wounds, early turning grey, weakened immune system	Old people, pregnant and nursing women, burden, drinking much coffee and tea	Water-soluble, heat-sensitive	approx. 10mg

Vitamin B6 (Pyridoxin)	Bananas, nuts, wholemeal products, yeast, liver, potatos, green beans, cauliflower, carrots	Travel sickness, neuralgia, liver damage, premenstrual syndrome, digestion of protein, most important hormone in pregnancy together with folic acid, detoxication	(Rather rarely) intestine problems, bad skin, tiredness, rough corners of the mouth	Period of growth, intake of birth control pill, cortisone, during physical and mental load, before menstruation	Water-soluble, neither heat nor light-resisting	approx. 2mg
Vitamin B7 (Biotin, Vitamin H)	Liver, cauliflower, champignons, wholemeal products, eggs, avocado, spinach, milk	Skin diseases, loss in growth of hairs, liver damage, assists metabolism, carbohydrate and fatty acid activity, together with vitamin K it is needed for building up the clotting factors	States of exhaustion, skin inflammations, muscular pains, hair loss, nausea	Intake of birth control pill, antibiotics and cathartics	Water-soluble	approx. 0.5mg
Vitamin B9 (Folic acid, Vitamin M)	Liver, wheat germs, cucurbit, champignons, spinach, avocado	Liver damage, cell division, healing and growth of muscles and cells, protein metabolism	Anaemia, digesting disturbances, disturbances of hair -, bone and cartilage growth	Pregnant and nursing women, smoker, youth	Water-soluble, do not tolerate with heat, light or oxygen	approx. 160µg
Vitamin B12 (Cobalamin)	Liver, milk, yolk, fish, meat, oysters, quark, barm	Building substance of cytoblast and erythrocyte, nerve pains, skin and mucosa inflammation, liver damage	Anaemia, nervous disturbances, changes in the lung and the spinal marrows	Diabetics, pregnant and nursing women, vegetarian, vegan, intake of birth control pill, antibiotics and anti-cramp means, chemotherapy	Water-soluble, heatproof	approx. 5µg
Vitamin C (ascorbic acid)	Dogroses, sea buckthorn, citric fruits, black currants, potatoes, paprika, tomatoes, collard, spinach, vegetables, radish	Inflammation and bleeding restraining, assists the body's defences, protects cells against chemical destruction, activates enzymes, structure of connective tissue, bones and dental enamel, faster healing of wounds, stabilisation of psyche	Gum-bleed, tiredness, joint pain and headache, bad healing of wounds, lack of appetite, scurvy, inefficiency	Smoker, pregnant and nursing women, older people, diets, alcohol consumption, intake of birth control pill, antibiotics, cortisone, analgesics and barbiturates	Water-soluble, oxygen and dryness-sensitively, not for a long time store	approx. 75-200mg

Vitamin D (Calciferol)	Cod-liver oil, liver, milk, yolk, butter, sea fish, herring, champignons, avocado	Regulation of calcium and phosphate, household, structure of bone, assists admission of calcium	Bone curvature and softening, increased infection, sensitivity, amyasthenia	Babies, older humans, intake of birth control pill, antibiotics, barbiturate	Fat-soluble, light sensitively, heatproof	approx. 5µg
Vitamin E (Tocopherole)	Sunflowers, corn , soya and wheat germ oil, nuts, flaxseed, salsify, peperoni, collard, avocado	Stabilization of the immune system, anti-inflammatory, cell replacement, protection from radicals, modulates cholesterol level and hormone household, important for blood vessels, muscles and reproduction organs	(Rarely) amblyopia, tiredness, amyotrohia, reproduction problems	intake of cathartics and blood-fat-lowering medicines, high consumption of alcohol	Fat-soluble, it is destroyed by open storage, deep-freezing or cooking with much fat	10-30mg (with fat-enrich nutrition more)
Vitamin K (Phyllochinone)	Eggs, liver, green collard, green vegetable, bulbs, oatmeal, kiwi fruit, tomatoes, cress	Necessary for formation of the blood clotting factors	High doses of vitamin A and E work against vitamin K.	Babies, high consumption of alcohol, intake of birth control pill, antibiotics and carthartics	Fat-soluble, food with Vitamin K should be stored darkly	approx. 2mg

Note: The 'Overdosing' column from the table can be seen by visiting the following Website:
http://jumk.de/bmi/vitamin-table.php#b3

222

Table 3: Minerals
Introduction and Summary Tables

Mineral	Chemical element (as opposed to organic compound, as in the case of vitamins) necessary for the health and maintenance of bodily functions
Macro Mineral	Definitions vary slightly from one source to another, but common definitions of macro minerals include: 1) minerals found in a typical adult human body in quantities greater than 5g. 2) Minerals required by a typical adult human body in quantities greater than 100mg per day.
Micro Mineral	Definitions vary slightly from one source to another, but common definitions of micro minerals include: 1) Minerals found in a typical adult human body in quantities less than 5g. 2)Minerals required by a typical adult human body in quantities of 1mg-100mg per day.
Trace Element	Chemical element (as opposed to organic compound, as in the case of vitamins) required in minute concentrations for normal bodily development and growth. There is some overlap between the classification of elements as "Micro Minerals" and "Trace Elements"; different textbooks favouring one or other category for elements such as copper, manganese, zinc and others. In case of "Trace Elements", of the two definitions stated above, (relating to the typical daily requirement) may be the most helpful because according to this definition Trace Elements are described as "Minerals required by a typical human body in quantities of less than 1mg per day". Examples of trace elements include: flourine, iodine, cobalt, molybdenum, silicon, and others.

Table 3: Minerals continued. Summary table: The following table (in alphabetical order within categories) includes basic information about some of the major minerals used by the human body.

Mineral	Functions	Sources	Signs of Deficiencies
Macro Minerals:			
Calcium (Ca)	Key constituent of bones and teeth; essential for vital metabolic processes such as nerve function, muscle contraction, and blood clotting.	Dairy produce	Deficiency (or insufficient uptake) may lead to: osteomalacia; osteoporosis; rickets; tetany.
Iron (Fe)	Essential for transfer of oxygen between tissues in the body.	Blood (e.g. "Black Pudding"); Eggs; Green (leafy) vegetables; Fortified foods (e.g. cereals, white flour); liver; meat; nuts; offal; peas; whole grains.	Deficiency may lead to: anaemia; increased susceptibility to infections.
Magnesium (Mg)	Essential for healthy bones; functioning of muscle & nervous tissue; needed for functioning of approx. 90 enzymes.	Eggs; Green leafy vegetables; fish (esp. shellfish); milk (and dairy products); nuts; wholemeal flour.	Deficiency can occur gradually, leading to: anxiety; fatigue; insomnia; muscular problems; nausea; premenstrual problems. The most extreme cases of deficiency may be associated with arrhythmia.
Phosphorous (P)	Constituent of bone tissue; forms compounds needed for energy conversion reactions e.g. adenosine triphosphate – (ATP).	Dairy products; fruits (most fruits); meat; pulses; vegetables(esp.leafy green).	Insufficient phosphorous may lead to: anaemia; demineralization of bones; nerve disorders; respiratory problems; weakness; weight Loss.
Potassium (K)	Main base ion of intracellular fluid; necessary to maintain electrical potentials of the nervous system - and so functioning of muscle and nerve tissues.	Cereals; coffee; fresh fruits; meat; salt-subsitutes; vegetables; whole-grain flour.	Insufficient potassium in the body may lead to: general muscle paralysis; metabolic disturbances.
Sodium (Na)	Controls the volume of extracellular fluid in the body; maintains the acid-alkali (pH) balance in the body; necessary to maintain electrical potentials of the nervous system - and so functioning of muscle and nerve tissues.	Processed bakery products; processed foods generally (incl. tinned and cured products); table salt	Insufficient sodium in the body may lead to: low blood pressure; general muscle weakness/paralysis; mild Fever; respiratory problems.
Micro Minerals:			
Chromium (Cr)	Involved in the functioning of skeletal muscle.	Cereals; cheese; fresh fruit; meat; nuts; wholemeal flour.	Deficiency may lead to: confusion; depression; irritability; weakness.

224

Copper (Cu)	Part of the enzyme copper-zince superoxide dismutase (CuZn SOD); Also present in other enzymes, including cytochrome oxidase, ascorbic acid oxidase, and tyrosinases; found in the red blood cells, and in blood plasma;	Cocoa; liver; kidney; oysters; peas; raisins.	Insufficient copper has been associated with: changes in hair colour & texture, and hair loss; disturbances to the nervous system; bone diseases. Serious deficiency is rare but can lead to: Menke's syndrome.
Manganese (Mn)	Antioxidant properties; fertility; formation of strong healthy bones, nerves, and muscles; forms part of the enzyme copper-zince superoxide dismutase (CuZn SOD) system;	Avocados; nuts; pulses; tea; vegetables; whole-grain cereals.	Deficiencies are unusual but may lead to: bone deformities; rashes & skin conditions; reduced hair growth; retarded growth (in children).
Selenium (Se)	Antioxidant properties (prevents peroxidation of lipids in the cells); Essential component of the enzyme glutathione peroxidase; Contributes to efficiency of the immune system - very wide variety of protective functions within the body.	Egg yolk; garlic; seafood; whole-grain flour.	Deficiency may lead to: cardiomyopathy; Kaschin-Beck disease (affects the cartilage at joints).
Sulphur (S)	Healing build-up of toxic substances in the body; structural health of the body (sulphur is a part of many amino acids incl. cysteine and methionine); healthy skin, nails & hair.	Beans; beef; cruciferous vegetables (e.g. broccoli); dairy produce; meat .	Deficiency of sulphur is unusual.
Zinc (Zn)	Needed for: functioning of many (over 200) enzymes; strong immune system;	Dairy produce; egg yolk; liver; red meat; seafood; whole-grain flour.	Deficiency is rare but may lead to: lesions on the skin, oesophagus and cornea; retarded growth (of children); susceptibility to infection.

http://www.ivy-rose.co.uk/Topics/Minerals.htm

225

Table 4: The Fibre Content of Some Foods. Approximate dietary fibre content of selected foods. Aim to eat at least one fibre-rich food at every meal or about 18 to 30grams of fibre per day.

Food	Average serving	Dietary fibre (g)
Breakfast cereals		
Shredded Wheat	1 medium-sized bowl (40g)	3.9g
Weetabix	2 Weetabix (37.5g)	3.9g
Shreddies	1 medium-sized bowl (40g)	3.8g
Fruit 'n' Fibre	1 medium-sized bowl (40g)	2.8g
Bread		
Granary bread	2 slices (70g)	3.0g
Brown bread	2 slices (70g)	2.5g
White bread	2 slices (70g)	1.1g
Pulses/vegetables		
Brussels sprouts	3 tablespoons (100g)	3.1g
Onions (fried in oil)	1 medium sized (100g)	3.1g
Broccoli (boiled)	2 tablespoons (75g)	2.3g
Carrots (boiled)	3 tablespoons (75g)	1.9g
Spinach (boiled)	3 tablespoons (120g)	1.9g
Fruit		
Pear (with skin)	1 medium sized (150g)	3.6 g
Avocado	1/2 medium sized (100g)	3.4g
Apple (with skin)	1 medium sized (150g)	3.1g
Orange	1 medium sized (160g)	2.7g
Banana	1 medium sized (200g)	2.2g
Peach (with skin)	1 medium sized (110g)	1.7g
Raspberries		1.5g
Strawberries	3 tablespoons (100g)	1.1g
Dried fruit/nuts		
Almonds	1 tablespoon (25g)	1.9g
Peanuts	1 tablespoon (25g)	1.6g
Mixed nuts	1 tablespoon (25g)	1.1g
Brazil nuts	1 tablespoon (25g)	1.1g
Other foods		
Spinach pakora/bhajia (fried)	50g	3.5g
Onion pakora/bhajia (fried)	50g	2.8g
Potato crisps (low fat)	1 small bag (35g)	2.2g

Table 5: Acid and Alkaline Forming Foods. This chart is intended only as a general guide to alkalizing and acidifying foods

...ALKALINE FOODS...	...ACIDIC FOODS...
ALKALIZING VEGETABLES	**ACIDIFYING VEGETABLES**
Alfalfa	Corn
Barley Grass	Lentils
Beet Greens	Olives
Beets	Winter Squash
Broccoli	
Cabbage	**ACIDIFYING FRUITS**
Carrot	Blueberries
Cauliflower	Canned or Glazed Fruits
Celery	Cranberries
Chard Greens	Currants
Chlorella	Plums**
Collard Greens	Prunes**
Cucumber	
Dandelions	**ACIDIFYING GRAINS, GRAIN PRODUCTS**
Dulce	Amaranth
Edible Flowers	Barley
Eggplant	Bran, oat
Fermented Veggies	Bran, wheat
Garlic	Bread
Green Beans	Corn
Green Peas	Cornstarch
Kale	Crackers, soda
Kohlrabi	Flour, wheat
Lettuce	Flour, white
Mushrooms	Hemp Seed Flour
Mustard Greens	Kamut
Nightshade Veggies	Macaroni
Onions	Noodles
Parsnips (high glycemic)	Oatmeal
Peas	Oats (rolled)
Peppers	Quinoa
Pumpkin	Rice (all)
Radishes	Rice Cakes
Rutabaga	Rye
Sea Veggies	Spaghetti
Spinach	Spelt
Spirulina	Wheat Germ
Sprouts	Wheat
Sweet Potatoes	

Tomatoes	**ACIDIFYING BEANS & LEGUMES**
Watercress	Almond Milk
Wheat Grass	Black Beans
Wild Greens	Chick Peas
	Green Peas
ALKALIZING ORIENTAL VEGETABLES	Kidney Beans
Daikon	Lentils
Dandelion Root	Pinto Beans
Kombu	Red Beans
Maitake	Rice Milk
Nori	Soy Beans
Reishi	Soy Milk
Shitake	White Beans
Umeboshi	
Wakame	**ACIDIFYING DAIRY**
	Butter
ALKALIZING FRUITS	Cheese
Apple	Cheese, processed
Apricot	Ice Cream
Avocado	Ice Milk
Banana (high glycemic)	
Berries	**ACIDIFYING NUTS & BUTTERS**
Blackberries	Cashews
Cantaloupe	Legumes
Cherries, sour	Peanut Butter
Coconut, fresh	Peanuts
Currants	Pecans
Dates, dried	Tahini
Figs, dried	Walnuts
Grapes	
Grapefruit	**ACIDIFYING ANIMAL PROTEIN**
Honeydew Melon	Bacon
Lemon	Beef
Lime	Carp
Muskmelons	Clams
Nectarine	Cod
Orange	Corned Beef
Peach	Fish
Pear	Haddock
Pineapple	Lamb
Raisins	Lobster
Raspberries	Mussels
Rhubarb	Organ Meats
Strawberries	Oyster
Tangerine	Pike

Tomato	Pork
Tropical Fruits	Rabbit
Umeboshi Plums	Salmon
Watermelon	Sardines
	Sausage
ALKALIZING PROTEIN	Scallops
Almonds	Shellfish
Chestnuts	Shrimp
Millet	Tuna
Tempeh (fermented)	Turkey
Tofu (fermented)	Veal
Whey Protein Powder	Venison
ALKALIZING SWEETENERS	**ACIDIFYING FATS & OILS**
Stevia	Avacado Oil
	Butter
ALKALIZING SPICES & SEASONINGS	Canola Oil
Chili Pepper	Corn Oil
Cinnamon	Flax Oil
Curry	Hemp Seed Oil
Ginger	Lard
Herbs (all)	Olive Oil
Miso	Safflower Oil
Mustard	Sesame Oil
Sea Salt	Sunflower Oil
Tamari	
	ACIDIFYING SWEETENERS
ALKALIZING OTHER	Carob
Alkaline Antioxidant Water	Corn Syrup
Apple Cider Vinegar	Sugar
Bee Pollen	
FRESH FRUIT JUICE	**ACIDIFYING ALCOHOL**
Green Juices	Beer
Lecithin Granules	Hard Liquor
Mineral Water	Spirits
Molasses, blackstrap	Wine
Probiotic Cultures	
Soured Dairy Products	**ACIDIFYING OTHER FOODS**
Veggie Juices	Ketchup
	Cocoa
ALKALIZING MINERALS	Coffee
Calcium: pH 12	Mustard
Cesium: pH 14	Pepper
Magnesium: pH 9	Soft Drinks
Potassium: pH 14	Vinegar

Sodium: pH 14	
	Aspirin
Although it might seem that citrus fruits would have an acidifying effect on the body, the citric acid they contain actually has an alkalinizing effect in the system.	Chemicals
	Drugs, Medicinal
Note that a food's acid or alkaline forming tendency in the body has nothing to do with the actual pH of the food itself. For example, lemons are very acidic, however the end products they produce after digestion and assimilation are very alkaline so, lemons are alkaline forming in the body. Likewise, meat will test alkaline before digestion, but it leaves very acidic residue in the body so, like nearly all animal products, meat is very acid forming.	Drugs, Psychedelic
	Herbicides
	Pesticides
	Tobacco
	ACIDIFYING JUNK FOOD
	Beer: pH 2.5
	Coca-Cola: pH 2
	Coffee: pH 4
http://home.bluegrass.net/~jclark/alkaline	

** These foods leave an alkaline ash but have an acidifying effect on the body.

230

Table 5a: Activities of Autonomic Nervous System

Visceral Effector	Effect of Sympathetic Stimulation	Effect of Parasympathetic Stimulation
Eye		
Iris	Contracts dilator muscle of iris and brings about dilation of pupil	Contracts sphincter muscle of iris and brings about constriction of pupil. Contracts ancillary muscle and accommodates lens for near vision
Ancillary muscle	No innervation	Contracts ancillary muscle and accommodates lens for near vision
Glands		
Sweat	Stimulates secretion	No innervation
Lacrimal (tear)	Vasoconstriciton, which inhibits secretion	Normal or excessive secretion
Salivary	Vasoconstriciton, which decreases salivary	Stimulation of salivary secretion
Gastric	Vasoconstriciton, which inhibits secretion	Secretion stimulated
Intestinal	Vasoconstriciton, which inhibits secretion	Secretion stimulated
Adrenal medulla	Promotes epinephrine and norepinephrine	No innervation
Adrenal cortex	Promotes glucocorticoid secretion	No innervation
Lungs (bronchial tubes)	Dilation	Constriction
Heart	Increases rate and strength of contraction; dilates coronary vessels that supply blood to heart muscle cells	Decreases rate and strength of contraction; constricts coronary vessels
Blood vessels		
Skin	Constriction	No innervation for most
Skeletal muscle	Dilation	No innervation
Visceral organs (except heart and lungs)	Constriction	No innervation for most
Liver	Promotes glycogenolysis; decreases bile secretion	Promotes glycogenesis; increases bile secretion
Stomach	Decreases motility	Increases motility
Intestines	Decreases motility	Increases motility
Kidney	Constriction of blood vessels that results in decreased urine volume	No innervation
Pancreas	Inhibits secretion	Promotes secretion

Spleen	Contraction and discharge of stored blood into general circulation	No innervation
Urinary bladder	Relaxes muscular wall; increases tone in internal sphincter	Contracts muscular wall; relaxes internal sphincter
Arrector pili of hair follicles	Contraction results in erection of hairs ("goose pimples")	No innervation
Uterus	Inhibits contraction if non-pregnant; stimulates contraction if pregnant	Minimal effect
Sex organs	In male, vasoconstricition of ductus deferens, seminal vesicle, prostate; results in ejaculation. In female, reverse uterine peristalsis	Vasoldilation and erection in both sexes; secretion in female
(Tortora G J, 1983)		

Table 6: Digestive Enzymes

Enzyme	Glandular Source	Site of Action and pH	Substrate or food acted upon	Product
Salivary amylase	Salivary Glands (Mouth)	Mouth neutral (7)	Starch	Maltose
Pepsin	Gastric Glands (Stomach)	Stomach acidic (3.5)	Proteins	Peptides
Pancreatic amylase	Pancreas	Small intestine basic (7.5)	Starch	Maltose
Trypsin	Pancreas	Small intestine basic (7.5)	Protein	Peptides
Lipase	Pancreas	Small intestine basic (7.5)	Fat droplets	Glycerol and fatty acids
Nulease	Pancreas and small intestine	Small intestine basic (7.5)	Nucleic acids (DNA & RNA)	Nucleotides
Peptidases	Small intestine	Small intestine	Peptides	Amino acids
Maltase	Small intestine	Small intestine basic (7.5)	Maltose	Glucose
Nucleosidases	Small intestine	Small intestine basic (7.5)	Nucleotides	Base, sugar, phosphate

http://www.coolschool.ca/lor/BI12/unit8?U08L02.htm

Table 7: The Barnes Axillary Temperature Test

Patient's name: Starting date:

°C		°F
37.2		99.0
37.1		98.8
37.0		98.6
36.9		98.4
36.8		98.2
36.7		98.0
36.6		97.8
36.5		97.6
36.4 *		97.4
36.3		97.2
36.2		97.0
36.1		96.8
36.0		96.6
35.9		96.4
35.8		96.2
35.7		96.0
35.6		95.8
35.5		95.6

Day

*   If below, then hypothyroid

Table 8: Protein Content of Selected Vegan Foods. This table shows the amount of protein in various vegan foods and also the number of grams of protein per 100 calories. To meet protein recommendations, the typical adult male vegan needs only 2.5 to 2.9 grams of protein per 100 calories and the typical adult female vegan needs only 2.1 to 2.4 grams of protein per 100 calories. These recommendations can easily be met from vegan sources.

Food	Amount	Protein (g)	Protein (g/100 cal)
Tempeh	1 cup	41	9.3
Seitan	3 oz	31	22.1
Soybeans, cooked	1 cup	29	9.6
Lentils, cooked	1 cup	18	7.8
Black beans, cooked	1 cup	15	6.7
Kidney beans, cooked	1 cup	13	6.4
Veggie burger	1 patty	13	13.0
Chickpeas, cooked	1 cup	12	4.2
Veggie baked beans	1 cup	12	5.0
Pinto beans, cooked	1 cup	12	5.7
Black-eyed peas, cooked	1 cup	11	6.2
Tofu, firm	4 oz	11	11.7
Lima beans, cooked	1 cup	10	5.7
Quinoa, cooked	1 cup	9	3.5
Tofu, regular	4 oz	9	10.6
Bagel	1med. (3oz)	9	3.9
Peas, cooked	1 cup	9	6.4
Textured vegetable protein (TVP), cooked	1/2 cup	8	8.4
Peanut butter	2 tbsp	8	8.4
Veggie dog	1 link	8	13.3
Spaghetti, cooked	1 cup	8	3.7
Almonds	1/4 cup	8	3.7
Soy milk, commercial, plain	1 cup	6	4.0
Soy yoghurt, plain	6 oz	6	4.0
Bulgur, cooked	1 cup	6	3.7
Sunflower seeds	1/4 cup	6	3.3
Whole wheat bread	2 slices	5	3.9
Cashews	1/4 cup	5	2.7
Almond butter	2 tbsp	5	2.4
Brown rice, cooked	1 cup	5	2.1
Spinach, cooked	1 cup	5	13.0
Broccoli, cooked	1 cup	4	6.8
Potato	1 medium (60z)	4	2.7
Reference: USDA Database for Standard Reference, Release 18, 2005			

Table 8a: Food Additives (some of the most frequently used): Functions and Effects

E Number	Name	Function	Examples of Some Typical Products	Comments	Effects Reported in Sensitive People
E 100	Curcumin	Colour	Ice cream, edible fats and oils, confectionery	From turmeric, using methanol, hexane and acetone during processing	No adverse effects known with normal use. Excessive use in pigs caused thyroid cells to increase and multiply abnormally
E 102	Tartrazine	Colour, azo dye	Soft drinks, ice cream, confectionery, smoked fish, biscuits, medicine capsules, skin-care products	Prohibited in Norway and Austria	Migraine headaches, asthma, urticaria, rhinitis, wakefulness in children. Hyperactive Children's Support Group (HCSG) recommend eliminate from diet
E 104	Quinoline yellow	Colour, coal tar or azo dye	Confectionery, soft drinks, smoked fish, scotch eggs	Prohibited in Norway, USA, Australia, Japan	HCSG recommend eliminate from diet
E 110	Sunset yellow	Colour, azo dye	Confectionery, yoghurt, bread crumbs, jam, hot chocolate, packet soups, desserts and drinks	Prohibited in Norway, Sweden, Finland	Urticaria, angioedema (swelling on skin), gastric upset, vomiting. HCSG recommend eliminate from diet
E 122	Carmosine	Colour, azo dye	Confectionery, yoghurts, icecreams, jams, drinks, sauces, brown sauce	Prohibited in Norway, Sweden, USA, Japan	Urticaria, oedema. HCSG recommend eliminate from diet
E 123	Amaranth	Colour, azo dye	Confectionery, fruit pie fillings, desserts, soups, gravy mixes	Prohibited in Norway, restricted in France, Italy	Caused malignant tumours in rats. Urticaria. HCSG recommend eliminate from diet
E 124	Ponceau or cochineal red	Colour, azo dye	Confectionery, desserts, meat paste, soup	Prohibited in Norway, USA	Asthma
E 127	Erythrosine	Colour, coal tar or azo dye	Glace cherries, custard mix, desserts, tinned meat, dental plaque tablets	Prohibited in Norway, USA	Large amounts may increase thyroid activity and tumours. USA banned as being carcinogenic. Implicated in minimal brain dysfunction in children. Can cause phototoxicity (sensitivity to light)
E 128	Red 2G	Colour, azo dye	Sausages, meat products, jams, drinks	Prohibited in Norway, Sweden, Finland, Austria, USA, Canada, Japan, Switzerland, Australia	Can contribute to anaemia through its interference with haemoglobin. HCSG recommend eliminate from diet

E Number	Name	Function	Examples of Some Typical Products	Comments	Effects Reported in Sensitive People
E 131	Patent blue	Colour, coal tar or azo dye	Scotch eggs		Skin sensitivity, itching, urticaria, shock, breathing problems, nausea, low blood pressure, tremor. HCSG recommend eliminate from diet
E 132	Indigo carmine	Colour, coal tar or azo dye	Confectionery, meat products, gravy mixes	Prohibited in Norway	Nausea, vomiting, high blood pressure, skin rashes, itching, breathing problems. May cause sensitivity to viral diseases, HCSG recommend eliminate from diet
E 133	Brilliant blue	Colour, coal tar or azo dye	Confectionery, tinned peas, cosmetics, bacon, flavoured snacks	Prohibited in Austria, Belgium, Denmark, France, Greece, Italy, Spain, Switzerland, Norway, Sweden, Germany	HCSG recommend eliminate from diet
E 142	Green	Colour	Confectionery, tinned peas, packet bread crumbs, mint jelly, lime drinks	Prohibited in Norway, Sweden, Finland, Japan, Canada, USA	Very large amounts show weight gain, mild anaemia, mild thyroid degeneration in rats
E 150	Caramel	Colour	Some drinks (e.g. cola, whisky, brandy, beer) gravy, soups, sauces, bread, vinegar, beef products, confectionery, desserts	Produced from sugar	Some types of caramel colour (there are four) may cause gastro-intestinal symptoms, including diarrhoea
E 151	Black PN	Colour, azo dye	Fruit and brown sauces, cheesecakes, chocolate mousse	Prohibited in Norway, Finland, Japan, USA, Canada	Caused intestinal cysts in pigs. HCSG recommend eliminate from diet
E 154	Brown FK	Colour, azo dye	Crisps, cooked ham, kippers, smoked fish	Prohibited in USA, Finland, Norway, Sweden, Canada, Japan, Australia, France, Belgium, Spain, Portugal, Greece, Ger-many, Holland	Can cause genetic mutation, degeneration of skeletal, heart and general muscle damage. Link to salmonella, may be carcinogenic. HCSG recommend eliminate from diet

E Number	Name	Function	Examples of Some Typical Products	Comments	Effects Reported in Sensitive People
E 155	Brown HT	Colour, azo dye	Chocolate-flavour cakes, processed food	Prohibited as above	Asthma, skin sensitivity. HCSG recommend eliminate from diet
E 160a	Beta-carotene	Colour	Tinned soup, soft drinks, salad cream, milk products, margarine, infant food	Laboratory manufactured, extracted from carrots using hexane	Those with cancer have been found to be low in beta-carotene/vitamin A. Not known if this is cause or result of cancer
E 171	Titanium dioxide	Colour	Confectionery, some cheeses, toothpaste, horseradish sauce, sunscreen, gelatine capsules, make-up, paint, ink, filler for paper and plastic	Prohibited in Germany	No adverse effects known
E 202	Potassium sorbate	Preservative	Soft drinks, cakes, pre- packed sandwiches, milk products, wine		No adverse effects known
E 210	Benzoic acid	Preservative	Jam, beer, salad cream, margarine, manufacture of sodium benzoate, plasticizers, dyes, pharmaceuticals, soft drinks, sauces, syrups	Can inhibit digestive enzymes and glycine	Asthma, urticaria, gastric irritation, neurological disorders. HCSG recommend eliminate from diet
E 211	Sodium benzoate	Preservative	Soft drinks, salad dressings, sauces, prawns, sweets, body/mouth wash, shampoo		Asthma, urticaria. HCSG recommend eliminate from diet
E 212	Potassium benzoate	Preservative	Margarine, pickles, concentrated pineapple juice		As E 211
E 219	Hydroxyben-zoate salts	Preservative	Beer, cooked repacked beetroot coffee/chicory essence, flavouring, syrups, fruit pie fillings, soft drinks, pickles, sauces, snack meals	Produced from benzoic acid	Can cause skin reactions when applied externally or taken internally. Can have numbing effect on mouth. HCSG recommend eliminate from diet
E 222	Sodium hydrogen sulphite	Preservative	Instant potato, wine, beer, used on salads/ vegetables to prevent browning, used as a bleaching agent, fish, sugar, milk products, prawns		Linked to deaths of asthmatics in USA, may cause gastric irritation, skin reactions. Reduces vitamin B1 content of foods. HCSG recommend eliminate from diet

E Number	Name	Function	Examples of Some Typical Products	Comments	Effects Reported in Sensitive People
E 223	Sodium metabisul-phate	Preservative	Lemon juice, pickles, squash, carton salad, prawns, dried fruit/nuts, alcohol, home brewing		Asthma, skin reactions, gastric irritation, those with impaired kidneys or liver should avoid sulphites. Reduces vitamin B1 contents of foods. HCSG recommend eliminate from diet
E 250	Sodium nitrite	Preservative	Cooked, cured, tinned meat products	Also dyestuffs and corrosion inhibitor in industry	Can affect oxygen in blood, resulting in difficult breathing, pallour, dizziness, headaches. Potentially carcinogenic. HCSG recommend eliminate from diet
E 251	Sodium nitrite	Preservative	Cooked, cured meat, some cheeses		As E 250
E 252	Potassium nitrate	Preservative	For curing and preserving meat		May cause anaemia, kidney inflammation, gastroenteritis, severe abdominal pain, vomiting, muscular weakness, irregular pulse. Potentially carcinogenic
E 260	Acetic acid	Acidity regulator	Pickles, cough mixture, rheumatic liniment, skin applications, fumes from silicone curing, all vinegars	Found naturally in plant and animal tissue, helps fatty acid-carbohydrate metabolism	No toxicological problems known
E 270	Lactic acid	Acidulant	Meat extracts, margarine, manufacture of bread additives, soft drinks, tinned food, baby milks, sports drinks, skin lotions, used in textile and leather finishing	Found naturally in muscles during physical exertion	May be difficult for babies to metabolise. No toxological problems for adults
E 296	Malic acid	Preservative	Commercial malic acid found in soft drinks, fruit pie fillings, cereal bars, tinned fruit, veg	Found naturally in fruit and veg	Not to be given to infants as not known whether infants can metabolise D-form of malic acid
E 300	Ascorbic acid vitamin C	Antioxidant	Softdrinks, bread, mustard, instant potato, tinned fruit, preserves, beer, wine	Chemically synthesised using glucose	Large doses can cause diarrhoea or dental erosion. More than 10g daily could result in kidney stones

E Number	Name	Function	Examples of Some Typical Products	Comments	Effects Reported in Sensitive People
E 320	Butylated hydro-xyanisole	Antioxidant	Confectionery, raisins, stock cubes, soft drinks, packet foods, potato snacks, mayonnaise, breakfast cereals, mascara	Prohibited for food use in Japan	High levels may promote mouth, throat, gullet cancers. May cause imbalance in fat metabolism. Not permitted in baby food. HCSG recommend eliminate from diet
E 321	Butylated hydro-xyanisole	Antioxidant	Body/face wash, perfume, blusher, mascara, shaving cream, margarines, veg oils, salted peanuts, gravy, packet foods, breakfast cereals		Skin rashes. Conflicting evidence whether it increases liver size, carcinogenic cell changes and reproductive failure. Not permitted in foods for children. Four grams a day causes cramps, weakness, nausea, vomiting, dizziness, loss of consciousness. NCSG recommend eliminate from diet
E 322	Lecitihin	Emulsifier	Confectionery, gravy granules, cakes, margarine, instant powdered products		No adverse effects known
E 330	Citric acid	Acidity regulator	Soft-drinks, jams, jellies, confectionery, mustard, sauces, tinned, packaged foods, cough mixtures, shampoo, body wash	Manufactured by the action of *Aspergillus niger* moulds of sugar	Has irritant action. Large amounts may erode teeth. (Bridget Main has found within her patient group that it can irritate skin, eyes, bladder, joints, behaviour in children)
E 331	Sodium citrate	Sequestrant (a chemical binder that prevents formation of clogging in some milk products)	Jams, jellies, soft drinks, confectionery, milk products, shampoo		Can alter urinary excretion of drugs, making them either less effective, or more toxic
E 334	Tartaric acid	Sequestrant	Jams, cakes, baking powder, confectionery, fizzy drinks, tinned food, tomato concentrates		Large amounts have laxative effect, may be mildly irritant or cause gastroenteritis
E 338	Phosphoric acid	Acidulent	Softdrinks, cooked meats, cocoa products, fats, oils, beer, rust remover		No adverse effects are known in food concentrations

240

E Number	Name	Function	Examples of Some Typical Products	Comments	Effects Reported in Sensitive People
E 400	Alginic acid	Stabiliser	Icecream, cheese, milkshakes, glazes, fish and meat, fruit juice, foam on beer, medicines, dressing on textiles	From brown seaweed	No known toxological risks
E 401	Sodium alginate	Stabiliser, suspending and thickening, gelling agent	Milk products, cakes, cereal bars, fruit juice, sauces, foam on beer	From brown seaweed	As E 400
E 407	Carageenan	Stabiliser, emulsifier, thickener, gelling agent	Ice-cream, salad dressings, jellies, desserts, reformed meat, toothpaste, shaving cream	'Irish Moss' seaweed	Large regular amounts have not shown to be totally safe, possible link to ulcerative colitis, and changes in mucous membranes
E 410	Locust bean gum	Stabiliser, emulsifier, thickener, gelling agent	Ice-cream, soft cheese, syrups, pie fillings, confectionery, sausages, tinned vegetables, tinned fish	From Carob tree	Effects unknown. Large amounts may inhibit absorption of nutrients
E 412	Guar gum	Stabiliser, thickener, emulsifier	Ice-cream, salad dressings, milk shakes, savoury sauces, tinned chicken, packet soups	From seeds of Indian pea family	Large amounts can cause nausea, flatulence, abdominal cramps, and inhibit absorption of nutrients
E 414	Gum acacia	Stabiliser thickener emulsifier	Soft-drinks, fruit gums, gateau mix, wine, beer, emulsifying/suspending agent in drugs, manufacture of plasters, as an adhesive	From Acacia tree	A few people have shown hypersensitivity after breathing it in, or eating it. Generally considered safe without adverse effects
E 415	Xanthan gum	Stabiliser thickener emulsifier	Soft-drinks, salad dress-ings, mustard, sauces, pickles, hot chocolate drinks, cereal bars, face lotions, toothpaste	Corn sugar gum	No adverse effects reported
E 420 (a)	Sorbitol	Sweetener	Low-calorie foods, con-fectionery, medicines, toothpaste, cosmetics, adhesives, polyurethane foams (Sorbitol is converted into sugar in the bloodstream, absorbed slowly, so useful source of sugar for diabetics)	Naturally in Rowan berries	Large amounts can cause flatulence, abdominal distension, or laxative effect. Not permitted in infant food

E Number	Name	Function	Examples of Some Typical Products	Comments	Effects Reported in Sensitive People
E 440 (a)	Pectin	Stabiliser, emulsifier, thickener, gelling agent	Jams, jellies, biscuits, desserts, salad dressings, cosmetics, laxatives	From rind of citrus fruits and apples, present in all plants	Large amounts may cause flatulence or intestinal distension
E 466	Sodium carboxy methylcel-lulose	Stabiliser, thickener, gelling agent	Icecream, cakes, soft drinks, toothpaste, suspending/dispersing agent in drugs	Made by treating cellulose from wood pulp	No adverse effects reported
E 491	Sorbitan monostea-rate	Emulsifier, stabiliser, glazing agent	Dried yeast, cakes, desserts, liquid tea concentrates		No adverse effects known
E 500	Sodium bicarbonate	Raising agent	Biscuits, cakes, antacids, beer making		No adverse effects in small doses, but large amounts can corrode gut, cause gastric upsets and circulation problems. Laboratory animals treated with it for lactic acidosis died more quickly/frequently than untreated animals. It has been recommended that its use in hospitals stops
E 621	Monosodium glutamate (MSG)	Flavour enhancer	Savoury snacks, pre-packed foods, meats, soups, tinned food, miso, tamari	From sugar or seaweed prohibited in baby food in USA	'Chinese restaurant syndrome': tightening muscles, numbness, nausea, stomach pains, palpitations, dizziness, cold sweat. Brain damage in animal tests
E 903	Carnuba wax	Glazing, polishing agent	Confectionery, furniture polish and varnish, mascara, depilatories, deodorant sticks	From leaves of Brazilian wax palm	Infrequently skin sensitivity or irritation
E 951	Aspartame	Artificial sweetner	Soft and fizzydrinks, low-calorie foods, confectionery, Canderel, NutraSweet		Considered a poison by many researchers and scientists stating aspartame changes to formaldehyde in the body
E 954	Saccharin	Artificial-sweetener	Soft, and fizzydrinks, low calorie foods, toothpaste, 'Sweet 'N Low'	Prohibited in Canada	Safety questioned in USA, digestive problems, carcinogenic, especially of bladder

E Number	Name	Function	Examples of Some Typical Products	Comments	Effects Reported in Sensitive People
Without E number classification	Dimethyl dicarbonate DMDC	Preservative	Softdrinks, fruit juices, wine		Potential irritant if inhaled, ingested, or on skin contact. Over-exposure = death. European Commission stated toxicology OK in drinks
Without E number classification	Oxalic acid	To produce antibiotics	Tea, coffee, chocolate, peanuts, spinach, beetroot, rhubarb	In many vegetables, some protein foods derived from vitamin C	May contribute to formation of kidney stones
Without E number classification	Vanillin	Flavour	Chocolate, cakes, yoghurt, perfume, cleaning products	From coniferyl alcohol (an organic compound) most synthetically made	
Without E number classification	Wood distillate	Used in the smoking of food - preservative	Smoke-flavour foods	Wood liquid (various types of wood), some may be carcinogenic hydrocarbons, creosote, camphor, acetone, dyes, wood oils, tar, Witch Hazel	

References: Researched and collated by Bridget Main 2007 (see useful addresses). Also see Davies S and Stewart A, 'Nutritional Medicine', Pan Books, 1987. Hanssen, M Marsden J 'E for Additives' Thorsons 1984.

Azo dyes – often those sensitve to asprin are sensitive to azo dyes, also those who suffer from asthma, eczema, urticaria, watery eyes/nose, oedema, blurred vision, in extreme cases can cause shock

Table 9: After Treatment Self-Care

You know that when old waste matter and toxins are disturbed they inevitably return to the bloodstream for elimination, or are prepared for evacuation by the bowel, when this is happening **the cleansing of your system has truly begun!** Your colon hydrotherapy treatment may stimulate, in the next few hours, several bowel movements. However, these will not be sudden, uncontrollable, or painful. Rather, it will be the colon performing its function of eliminating waste efficiently. Sometimes, when the colon is weak or sluggish there may be no bowel movement for several days. This is a likely indication that further treatments may be necessary alongside other aspects of your treatment plan. The removal of toxins can cause symptoms similar to feeling unwell, but remember the distinction between disease and healing is that **healing is the releasing of problems associated with, and from, your past,** a necessary part of your detoxification.

Suggestions for self-care

- After treatment try to avoid rushing around; try to find time to relax and to care for you. This is now **your time.**
- Enjoy a warm drink of peppermint tea or camomile tea, and rest.
- If you feel bloated or have wind pain have a drink of warm water and gently massage your stomach.
- Clearly avoid energetic exercise and movement as this may cause some discomfort.
- Allow your body to find 'quiet'.
- Listen to body, and when you feel ready, resume your normal meal-times.
- Make intelligent choices about food and consume only moderate amounts.
- Think about and consume that which you feel to be gentle and nourishing.
- You may choose a light meal of salad or fish, soup or vegetable juices, vegetables and fruit.
- At this stage avoid a heavy high-protein meal, and whatever you decide do not 'fill-up.'
- Avoid alcohol and if possible processed foods.
- Remember to take your probiotics in order to supplement your friendly bacteria.
- **You know that if you have any real difficulties you can telephone me for support and advice.**

Table 10: Treatment Consent Form

Name: ....

Freely give my consent to receive colon hydrotherapy treatment and accept full responsibility for that decision.

I have informed my Therapist of any medical conditions which I believe may affect my treatment. I understand that colon hydrotherapy is part of an overall approach to diet and lifestyle, and that it is not a medical treatment.

I have been made aware of the medical conditions which are contraindicated with colon hydrotherapy and that these include the following:

- Recent surgery to the rectum or abdomen (less than eight weeks)

- Blood pressure above 160/100

- Pregnancy (between three to eight months)

- Heart disease, kidney disease, liver/gall bladder disease

- Anaemia

- Severe haemorrhoids

- Fissures or fistulas

- Cancer of the bowel, rectum, liver, or kidney

- Abdominal hernia

- Bowel perforation

- Long-term oral steroid use

- I have also informed my Therapist that to my knowledge, I am not allergic to latex gloves

Signature: ....   Date: ....

Table 11: Colon Hydrotherapy Consultation Form

STRICTLY PRIVATE and CONFIDENTIAL

Name: .... Contact Telephone No.: ....
Address: ....
Reasons for consultation: ....
Medical conditions and/or past surgery: ....
Any contraindications Noted: ....

Blood pressure: ....
Current medication, if any, and why: ....
If any pain, please describe: ....
How often do you open your bowel per day, days, week? ....
Do you feel empty afterwards? ....
Is it easy to pass and what is the shape and consistency? ....

LIFESTYLE:

Aspects I value: ....
Aspects I wish were different: ....
Aspects I wish to change: ....
Exercise: ....

DIET:

Breakfast: ....
Lunch: ....
Dinner: ....
Snacks: ....
Are there foods you avoid? ....
Are there foods you eat daily? ....
Are there foods you may find difficult to give up? ....
Alcohol consumption per week: ....
Coffee/tea daily: ....

Tick: Non-smoker ☐   Smoker ☐   How many daily? ....

Which supplement/s, if any, are you taking, and please give reason/s:
....
....
....
....
....

Table 12: Treatment Plan Pro-forma

COLON HYDROTHERAPY TREATMENT PLAN RECORD

Name: ....

Date: ....

Reported Symptoms: ....

....

(Constipation, diarrhoea, gas, bloating, bowel noise, belching, flatulence, arthritis, acne, thrush, cystitis, *candida*, parasites, acne, fatigue, aching limbs, halitosis, PMT, any swelling, sleep disturbance/difficulties, cravings, water retention, pain, congestion, headaches, etc.)

Colon Hydrotherapy Procedure:

Duration: ....   Water pressure: ....   Temperature: ....

Massage: ....   ICV: ....

Rapport: ....

Notes: ....

....

Stool colour: ....   Consistency: ....   Quantity (0 to 10):...........

Blood: ....   Fats: ....   Wind: ....

Undigested food: ....   Discomfort: ....   Other:

Notes: ....

Lifestyle Adjustments:

Issues discussed: ....

Actions/changes (exercise, routines, stress management, squatting, timing, sleep preparation, supplements, etc.)

Agreed (the what): ....

Implementation strategy (the when, and how): ....

....

Dietary Issues:

Issues discussed: ....

Actions/changes (water, dietary changes/routines, fibre, chewing, food choices, 'addictions', allergy, eliminating possible symptom causes, etc.)

Agreed (the what): ....

Implementation strategy (the when, and how): ....

....

Nutritional Advice:

Detail: ....

Supplements issued: ....

Case Notes: ....

....

....

The Essential Reading and Reference Book List

(The following is the beginning of the colon hydrotherapist's library)

Essential Reading List:

Budd M.	**Why Am I So Tired?**	ISBN 0 7225 3942 8
Jacobs J.	**Beat Candida Through Diet**	ISBN 0 09 181545 2
Jensen B.	**Dr Jensen's Guide to Better Bowel Care**	ISBN 089529 284 9
Turner R.N.	**Naturopathic Medicine**	ISBN 0 9539151 0 7

Essential Reference List:

Brewer S.	**Encyclopaedia, of Vitamins, Minerals, and Herbal Supplements**	ISBN 1 84119 184 1
Holford P.	**New Optimum Nutrition Bible**	ISBN 0 7499 2552 3
Lindlahr H.	**Philosophy of Natural Therapeutics**	ISBN 0 85207 159 0
	Oxford Concise Medical Dictionary	ISBN 978 0 19860753.3
Tortora G. and Anagnostakos N.	**Principles of Anatomy and Physiology**	ISBN 0 06 046704 5

Useful Contacts and Addresses

1. Association of Natural Medicine, www.associationnaturalmedicine.co.uk

2. Association and Register of Colon Hydrotherapists, www.colonic-association.org/

3. Bridget Main, Food and Environmental Intolerance Testing and Homoeopathic Treatment, 01376 570067

4. British College of Naturopathy and Osteopathy, www.bcom.ac.uk/

5. Cathy Wong, www.altmedicine.about.com

6. College of Naturopathic Medicine, www.naturopathy-uk.com

7. David Goddard, Naturopath, 01621 816089

8. Digestive Disorders Foundation, www.corecharity.org.ukcoeliac.uk , www.coeliac.co.uk

9. Dotolo, www.colontherapysupplies.co.uk

10. Dr Hulda Clark, Research Association, www.drclark.com

11. Elizabeth Hughes, Kinesiologist, www.elizabethhughes.net

12. General Council and Register of Naturopaths, www.naturopathy.org.uk

13. Guild of Colon Hydrotherapists, www.colonic-association.com

14. *Herrmann Apparatebau* GmbH, (The Colon-Hydromat), www.h-a-b-gmbh.de/

15. Hydromat UK contact person is Pauline Gammon, The Specula Company, 01376 520438

16. Medicine Net, www.medicinenet.com

17. National Association for Colitis and Crohn's Disease, www.nacc.org.uk/

18. National Health Service Health Encyclopaedia, www.nhs.uk

19. National Health Service, National Electronic Library for Health, www.nelp.nhs.uk

20. Nelson Brunton, Naturopathic Doctor, acupuncturist, Natural Healing Centre 01376 511069

21.   Protein Content of Selected Vegan Foods, www.vrg.org

22.   Scottish School of Colonic Hydrotherapy, www.colonictraining.co.uk

23.   South Beach Diet and Glycaemic Index Food Chart, www.southbeach-diet

24.   Sources of Fibre, www.indiadiets.com/foods

25.   Transcom, www.transcomsl.com

26.   United Kingdom Gout Society, www.ukgoutsociety.org

27.   USDA Nutrient Database, www.nal.usda.gov/fnic/foodcomp/

28.   Women's Health, www.womenshealthlondon.org.uk

Bibliography

1.   Banerjee P N. **Chronic Disease, Its Cause and Cure**, B. Jain Pub., New Delhi 1931.

2.   Baroody T A. **Alkalize or Die**, Amazon, 2005.

3.   Bassler A. **Intestinal Toxaemia, Medical Journal and Record Vol. 136**, 1933.

4.   Bousvaros A. **Is There a Role for Probiotic Therapies in Inflammatory Bowel Disease?** Gastroenterology, Touch Briefings, 2008.

5.   Briel J W. et al., **'Clinical Value of Colonic Irrigation in Patients with Continence Disturbances'**, Department of General Surgery, University Hospital Dijkzigt, Rotterdam, The Netherlands: Dis Colon Rectum, 1997 Jul;40(7):802-5.

6.   Budd M. **Why Am I So Tired?** Thorsons, USA, 2000.

7.   Clark H C. **The Cure for all Diseases**, New Century Press, USA, 1995.

8.   Collings J. **Principles of Colonic Irrigation**, Thorsons, USA, 1996.

9.   DeFelice K L. **Enzymes: Go With Your Gut**, Amazon, 2006.

10.   Du Toit J et al. **Risk in Primary Care of Colorectal Cancer from New Onset Rectal Bleeding: 10 Year Prospective Study**, British Medical Journal, London, 2006.

11.   Freud S. **Beyond the Pleasure Principle**, Hogarth Press, London, 1920.

12.   Gloviezki P et al. **The Handbook of Venous Disorders**, American Venous Forum, USA, 2006.

13.   Hahnemann S. **Organon of Medicine**, Gollancz, London, 1989.

14.   Issels J. **Cancer – A Second Opinion**, Hodder and Stoughton, London, 1975.

15.   Iyengar B K S. **Light on Pranayama**, Unwin Paperbacks, UK, 1983.

16.   Jacobs G. **Beat Candida Through Diet**, Vermillion, London, 1997.

17.   Jensen B. **Tissue Cleansing Through Bowel Management**, BJ Enterprises, USA, 1981.

18.   Jensen B. **Dr. Jensen's Guide to Better Bowel Care**, Avery, USA, 1999.

19. Kellogg J H. **Colon Hygiene**, Good Health Publishing, Battle Creek, MI, 1916.

20. Kloss J K. **Back to Eden,** Back to Eden Pub. Co., USA, 1995.

21. Knight R. et al. **How to Practise Complementary Medicine Professionally**, Arima, Amazon, 2004.

22. Knight R. **A Guide to Helping Yourself and Others**, Cross-Roads Publications, Essex, England, 1992 (Association of Natural Medicine).

23. Kock S M. et al. **Colonic Irrigation**, International Journal of Colorectal Disease, 2008;23 (2):195-200.

24. Lindlahr H. **Philosophy of Natural Therapeutics**, C.W.Daniel Co. Ltd., England, 1975.

25. McGarey W A. **The Oil That Heals**, A.R.E. Press, 1999.

26. McHugh P. et al. **Buteyko Breathing Technique for Asthma and effective intervention**, New Zealand Medical Journal, 2003.

27. Food and Nutrition Board, Institute of Medicine. **Dietary Reference Intakes for Energy, Carbohydrate, Fibre, Fat, Fatty Acids, Cholesterol, Protein, and Amino Acids**, 2002.

28.   **Oxford Concise Medical Dictionary**, Oxford University Press, 2003.

29.   Requena Y. **Character and Health: The Relationship of Acupuncture and Psychology**, Paradigm Publications, 1989.

30.   Schiff J L. **Cathexis Reader**, Harper and Row, USA, 1975.

31.   The Department of Health, **National Diet and Nutrition Survey, People Aged 65 Years and Over**, 1998.

32.   The Department of Health, **Nutrition Action Plan**, 2007.

33.   Tortora G. and Anagnostakos N. **Principles of Anatomy and Physiology** (sixth edition), Harper Collins, USA, 1990.

34.   Turner R N. **Naturopathic Medicine, Treating the Whole Person, Health Advisory Lectures and Literature**, UK, 2000.

35.   Vassy C. **The Acid-Alkaline Diet**, Amazon, 2005.

36.   Walker N W. Colon Health, Norwalk Press, Arizona, 1979.

37.   Webster D. **Acidophilus and Colon Health**, Kensington Publishing Corps, New York, 1999.

38.   Weill A. **Eating Well for Optimum Health**, Time-Warner Paperbacks, UK, 2002.

39.   Weinberger S. **Healing Within: The Complete Guide to Colon Health**, Amazon, 1988.

Index

256

C

257

D

259

P

R

S

About the Author

Richard Knight has worked in the helping professions for 45 years as a practitioner, therapist, teacher, manager, trainer, lecturer, consultant, and in research and development. He holds professional qualifications in child care, education, art therapy, nutrition, and has successfully completed study of the theory and practice of colon hydrotherapy. His doctorate is in psychotherapy and counseling.

In 1983 Richard was a founder member of the Association of Natural Medicine, a Registered Charity, and for many years was its Vice President. He has run training courses nationally for central government departments, and other organisations, on the care and treatment of emotionally disturbed children and therapeutic interventions. Richard has shown, in his professional life and within complementary medicine, an unwavering commitment to the promotion and development of best practice, quality standards, informed professional judgement, and the empowerment of both the Helper and the Helpee in that search for increased self-awareness, individual autonomy, and wellbeing.

Notes

Notes

Notes

Notes

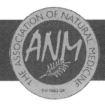
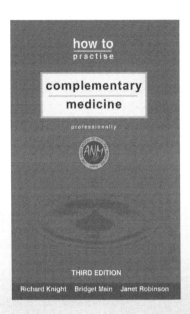

Lightning Source UK Ltd.
Milton Keynes UK
08 April 2011

170569UK00001B/6/P